'Nancy Stone's book comes at a critical time as societies around the world replace emotional relationship connections with wireless electronic messages and pieces of data. She gives examples of how midwifery education can identify therapeutic presence as the foundational essence of midwifery care and use it to turn birth into an empowering experience beyond the technology used, no matter what style of birth is chosen by the woman. The relational foundation of midwifery cannot be taught through texts or online modules. It needs to be experienced and felt and Stone gives us examples of how that can be modeled for students. Stone's use of stories from Greek mythology brings midwifery back to the humanities, demonstrating that the feelings that need to be recognized and nurtured for pregnancy and birth are timeless. Stone's book is a must read for midwifery teachers, practicing midwives, and student midwives.'

Cecilia M. Jevitt, *Professor, Midwifery Program,*
Director, University of British Columbia

'Dr. Nancy Stone's manuscript reveals the deep physiological wisdom embedded in relational caregiving. Her work thoughtfully integrates the lived experience of midwifery with the science of oxytocin and autonomic regulation. It affirms that birth and caregiving are not only clinical processes but relational neurobiological events—shaped by co-regulation, safety, and trust. This is a timely and meaningful contribution to the fields of reproductive health and human connection.'

Sue Carter, PhD, *Distinguished Research Professor,*
Emerita Director of the Kinsey Institute,
Indiana University, Professor of Psychology,
University of Virginia

'In this methodologically rigorous and beautifully articulated manuscript, Dr. Nancy Stone offers a compelling examination of midwifery in free-standing birth centres. Her focus on relational care and embodied knowledge reflects the core principles of Polyvagal Theory—particularly the role of co-regulation, neuroception, and the social transmission of safety. This work makes a significant contribution to our understanding of how caregiving environments shape autonomic regulation and support human resilience.'

Stephen W. Porges, PhD, *Originator of Polyvagal Theory,*
Distinguished University Scientist, founding
Director of the Kinsey Institute Traumatic Stress
Research Consortium, Indiana University,
Professor of Psychiatry,
University of North Carolina

'Nancy Stone has written the smartest, most thoughtful, most data-based discussion of the difference between midwifery in medical settings and midwifery as an independent profession.'

Barbara Katz Rothman, *Professor of Sociology, Public Health, Disability Studies and Women's Studies, City University of New York*

BECOMING A MIDWIFE IN A FREE-STANDING BIRTH CENTRE

This book explores the lived experiences of newly qualified midwives working in free-standing birth centres, highlighting the emotional, professional, and sociological aspects of their journeys from novices to confident practitioners in an out-of-hospital setting. As newly qualified midwives transition from their educational settings to the low-tech environment in their free-standing birth centre, they broaden their skill set, develop hands-on skills, and learn, for example, to care for labouring women without continuous fetal monitoring.

This book spotlights the skills needed to work in free-standing birth centres and the importance of becoming well integrated into a team, which, in turn, allows newly qualified midwives to build confidence in their abilities and offer comprehensive care to women and their families throughout pregnancy, birth, and the postpartum period. Capturing the skill acquisition, learning, and professional identity development of newly qualified midwives, this thoughtful book emphasises the critical role of mentorship from experienced midwives and the supportive environment for midwives and families in free-standing birth centres, many of which also offer home birth services.

This book is an essential contribution to the literature around midwifery practice, with an emphasis on physiological birth, continuity of care, skill acquisition, and professional identity development. It will be of use to students, practitioners, and scholars with an interest in these areas.

Nancy Iris Stone is an American-German midwife who has lived in Germany for nearly four decades. She has practised midwifery for 24 years in both hospital settings and a free-standing birth centre. Her research focuses on birth in free-standing birth centres, with particular attention to the lived experiences of women and birthing people, as well as midwives. Passionate about midwifery practice, she is committed to fostering the transmission of skills and knowledge between generations of midwives.

BECOMING A MIDWIFE IN A FREE-STANDING BIRTH CENTRE

"I am the midwife I dreamed of becoming"

Nancy Iris Stone

Routledge
Taylor & Francis Group

LONDON AND NEW YORK

Designed cover image: Nancy Stone

First published 2026
by Routledge
4 Park Square, Milton Park, Abingdon, Oxon OX14 4RN

and by Routledge
605 Third Avenue, New York, NY 10158

Routledge is an imprint of the Taylor & Francis Group, an informa business

For Product Safety Concerns and Information please contact our EU representative GPSR@taylorandfrancis.com. Taylor & Francis Verlag GmbH, Kaufingerstraße 24, 80331 München, Germany.

British Library Cataloguing-in-Publication Data
A catalogue record for this book is available from the British Library

ISBN: 978-1-032-96929-9 (hbk)
ISBN: 978-1-032-96928-2 (pbk)
ISBN: 978-1-003-59130-6 (ebk)

DOI: 10.4324/9781003591306

Typeset in Times New Roman
by codeMantra

For the midwives whose wisdom lives on in these and other stories, and for those still on the path of becoming. May this book be a companion to your journey.

CONTENTS

ABOUT THE AUTHOR

Nancy Iris Stone is an American-German midwife who has lived in Germany for nearly four decades. After qualifying as a midwife in 2001, she has worked across diverse settings, including hospital labour and delivery wards and a free-standing birth centre, and she is currently practising in a hospital-based midwifery team. She studied sociology and public health and obtained her PhD in Community Health and Midwifery from the University of Central Lancashire in 2019. Her research focuses on birth in free-standing birth centres, with particular attention to women's and midwives' lived experiences of pregnancy, labour, birth, and postpartum as critical knowledge for guiding midwifery practice and care. Passionate about midwifery practice, she is committed to fostering the transmission of skills and knowledge between generations of midwives.

FOREWORD

I am the midwife I dreamed of becoming: Developing relational care in midwifery practice

Soo Downe, Aug 29th 2025

"You have to trust in your hands and let the image take form."
(Nanette, Chapter 6, referring to abdominal palpation)

There are multitudes of papers published on outcomes of labour and birth in different settings. Volumes of books and book chapters describe the experiences of women and birthing people under various circumstances. In general, outcomes are at least as good in birth centres as in hospitals where pregnancy and labour are straightforward, and transfer arrangements are appropriate, seamless, and respectful. However, experiences of women using birth centres are often strikingly different from those of women who labour and give birth in hospitals. This has been explained by factors such as better staffing levels, more relaxed approaches to labour and birth progress, and different philosophies of care. None of these factors reveal the essence and meaning of the differences, and how they shape midwifery. What Nancy Stone has done in this book is to *let the image take form*.

She uses a delicate and intricate blend of phenomenology, myth, philosophy, and crafted stories based on midwives interviewed over time, from their first move from hospital to free-standing birth centre, up to a year later. As the text unfolds, these midwives become a lens through which the *habitus* of the birth centre emerges. The storytelling reveals how they gradually shed the stresses that had become literally embodied in them (written into their physical responses) through their hospital experiences. In the process, the reader becomes aware of the essential oddness of the way in which hospital labour and birth are currently conducted, without the text ever becoming a binary polemic about which place of birth is best. Over months of paying attention through observation as they become attuned to their changed environment, the newly qualified birth centre midwives slip from one way of seeing to another. They come to notice how the tension in their bodies and their previous default anxiety and hyper-alertness at work change into feelings of confidence and competence. They feel themselves becoming safe and joyful practitioners.

This text is not unrealistically idealistic. It also includes a story of a midwife who was deeply aligned with the philosophy of the birth centre, but who, despite months of mutual effort, could not become attuned to the birth centre team. This chapter demonstrates the critical value of a profound kind of relational group dynamic which is fundamental to safety, and which is not captured in the usual rhetoric of what 'teamwork' means.

Transfer is also addressed. The text shows that transfer between the birth centre and the hospital can be seamless, respectful, and part of a positive and triumphant labour and birth experience when handled well, whether the transfer is more or less of an emergency. Further, stories of midwives working with women who encounter stillbirth and intrauterine death acknowledge that, even in the best possible system with the best possible backup, sometimes tragedies happen. This book recognises the impact of this on those providing care, and how, in a relationship-rich, critically constructive environment, such experiences can be acknowledged as difficult, tragic, and profoundly moving, but also as a space for learning, rather than for blame, fear, and loss of confidence.

Although this book is originally designed for student midwives and midwives, it is also an important text for anyone who is interested in the meaning of midwifery and childbirth, and in the sociology and philosophy of maternity care more generally. It is a master class in how phenomenology and mythical symbolism can bring meaning into focus, opening a window into a deep understanding of the lifeworld of birth centre ways of being, and of the midwifery that is formed as a consequence. As Amelia (Chapter 13) says:

> This is where I'm at now. Out-of-hospital birth, like home birth or birth centre work, is always portrayed as so romantic and cozy—like those are the midwives who just love a comfy atmosphere but aren't clinically astute. And then hospital birth is framed as the tough stuff—the midwives who really know what they're doing, who are totally on the ball. And I was like, well, here I am, completely alone, in the middle of the night, responsible for two lives, and am completely aware of the clinical situation—managing it moment by moment AND I'm staying calm and gentle and am able to create this so-called "romantic atmosphere.". And I thought—what a funny contradiction. Those two things don't cancel each other out. Like, this really flips the script.

DATA AVAILABILITY STATEMENT

Due to the sensitive nature of this qualitative research and to protect participant confidentiality, the raw data cannot be shared in a public repository. However, extensive supporting data are included in this book and in related peer-reviewed publications.

AUTHOR'S NOTE

Throughout this book, I use the term *woman* when referring to those who are pregnant, giving birth, or in the postnatal period. This choice reflects the use of participant-driven language, preserving the terminology used by the midwives in the study whose lived experiences form the basis of this work. I acknowledge that pregnancy and birth are experienced by people of many gender identities, and that the term *woman* does not encompass the full diversity of those who give birth. My intention in retaining the language of the participants is to honour the authenticity and integrity of their voices.

ACKNOWLEDGEMENTS

I wish to thank the German Federal Ministry of Education and Research (BMBF) for funding my postdoctoral study *ASK a Midwife* (grant number 01GY2007), without which this book would not have been possible.

I am full of gratitude to the 15 newly qualified midwives who so generously shared their experiences with me. Their openness, thoughtfulness, and courage in the midst of transition brought this study to life. I would gladly work alongside each and every one of them. I am also deeply grateful to the experienced midwives who gave me their time and perspective; their reflections added depth and resonance, reminding me of how stories bind generations of midwives together.

I am indebted to the study's cooperating partners, who met with me twice a year to discuss preliminary study results and reflect on the significance of the study results from the perspective of their organisations: Anke Wiemer (Q.U.A.G. e.V.—Society for Quality in Out-of-Hospital Birth, Germany), Angelica Ensel (DGHWi—German Society of Midwifery Science), Christine Bruhn (Network of Free-Standing Birth Centres, Germany), and Maria Untsch (MotherHood e.V.).

Dorothea Tegethoff, one of my midwifery teachers over 25 years ago, encouraged me to pursue postdoctoral research, supported the development of the grant application, contributed input to publications, and joined meetings with the cooperating partners. Thank you! It has been a joy to come full circle in this way.

I am especially thankful to Gill Thomson for her sustained collaboration, scholarly insight, and for challenging me to read more deeply, write daily, and move beyond concepts and associations that limited my understanding. Her guidance made it possible to approach Heideggerian hermeneutic phenomenology with both rigour and confidence.

My thanks also go to my student assistant, Judith Krauleidies, who organised and supported so much of what goes on in the background of every study. I am also grateful to the Protestant University of Applied Sciences for providing an academic home during the project, and to Andrea Müller and Steven Suckow for their support in managing the finances.

I am also grateful to Barbara Katz Rothman, one of my earliest academic mentors, whose work and encouragement continue to shape my thinking. Heartfelt thanks to my friends Sara Sizer Marzona and Ellen Cassidy, who generously read parts of the manuscript and offered feedback that sharpened my writing. To my sister Linda, whose steady encouragement carried me through the long process of writing, and to my sister Sally, whose creativity and sensitivity as a writer continually remind me of the power of language.

Finally, I owe deepest gratitude to my partner, Bernd Oelmueller, who listened to my many stories of life on the road and on trains during the pandemic and helped me place this study within the wider world, beyond the birth centres and births themselves.

1

ASK A MIDWIFE

Acquisition of skills and knowledge of midwives in free-standing birth centres

In 2011, after completing my Master of Science in Public Health, I began working in a free-standing birth centre. I came with nine years of experience working in hospital labour and delivery wards with over 1,100 "catches" (births) and assumed that my orientation period would be brief before taking on full responsibility as the primary midwife at births. However, this was not the case. The owner and director of the birth centre, a midwife with over 40 years of experience, believed that hospital practice did not prepare a midwife for birth centre work. Because I had already spent three months observing and collecting data in a free-standing birth centre for my master's thesis, the director agreed to shorten my orientation period from the customary six months to three.

During my orientation there, my new colleagues often joked with me about what they called my "clinic reflexes." Those were moments where I was sure I had to "do" something, moments in which my colleagues continued to patiently observe. They noted that I moved around the room too much, made unnecessary suggestions, and had a restless twitch if the work pace felt too slow. During my three-month orientation period, in which I assisted the primary midwife at births, I learned to slow down and had time to reflect on my role and purpose as a midwife there, recognising the difference between disturbing and respecting, and distracting and facilitating. In building trusting relationships with clients, I began to understand how much information was passed between us that was unspoken and unquantifiable. Over time, I developed a profound appreciation for the work we did at the birth centre. I especially valued the opportunity to accompany our clients during pregnancy, labour, and birth, and to experience the benefits of continuity of care. In addition to this, my commitment to contribute to the study of midwifery in free-standing birth centres and home birth intensified.

DOI: 10.4324/9781003591306-1

I worked in the free-standing birth centre for nine years until it closed permanently in 2020 at the beginning of the COVID-19 pandemic. Directly after the closure, I started working in a hospital-based, independent midwifery team in the labour and delivery and postnatal wards. The relational quality of care that had become the foundation of my midwifery practice was suddenly, and profoundly, altered both by the change in setting and by the pandemic restrictions. One year into working in the hospital, a grant I had written was awarded by the German Federal Ministry of Education and Research (BMBF), grant number 01GY2007. The study was developed in collaboration with Gill Thomson (University of Central Lancashire) and Dorothea Tegethoff (University of Rostock), who both contributed to the preparation of the grant proposal. The study, entitled *ASK a Midwife*, was a hermeneutic phenomenology study, with the aim of gathering the lived experience of newly qualified midwives in their first year working in a free-standing birth centre. With this study, I wanted to fulfil a long-held goal to research the skills and knowledge that midwives need to develop when they commence work in free-standing birth centres. Gill Thomson, an expert in Heideggerian hermeneutic phenomenology and its use in qualitative health research, supported the analytic process and provided valuable scholarly input throughout.

I began collecting data after ethics approval in August 2021, when the COVID-19 pandemic was still impacting all aspects of our lives. I travelled by train throughout Germany to conduct interviews, focus groups, and rapid ethnography in free-standing birth centres and was often the only passenger in the carriage. Social distancing became a "thing" in that it was not just a rule, but a way in which the world re-gathered, affecting policy, physical space, and relationships. The pandemic foregrounded distance as a civic duty, while also revealing to me just how much I desperately missed the small interactions that had been a part of my daily life. A little over a year into the study, I boarded a train in which several carriages were out of service, forcing passengers to occupy every available seat. I quickly found a single seat sitting across from a woman who was in an online meeting. I tensed up as the other seats around me filled up, feeling vaguely uncomfortable, not because I was worried about getting COVID-19, but because of the overwhelming and now unfamiliar proximity to others. I found myself suddenly steeped in their presence in ways that I had taken for granted before the pandemic. We were connected through breath (albeit masked), voices, smells, and conversations. The atmosphere seemed charged with sounds and emotion.

On the train that day, I reflected on the interviews and data analysis that I had conducted up until that point and became deeply aware of the juxtaposition between the newly qualified midwives I was accompanying in their first year working in a free-standing birth centre and the person and midwife I had become during the pandemic. They were learning relational care and connection to others; I had learned to disconnect and distance myself from others. As I contemplated this, I began to grasp more fully the urgency of what the newly qualified midwives were learning in their orientation. In considering how quickly I had accepted the new normal of social distancing, I realised how exceptional it was to witness midwives learning empathic, embodied, and co-responsive care. The free-standing birth centres I visited during the study followed the pandemic restrictions and yet were oases of humanity and connection, continuing throughout to offer families a protected space to give birth.

History of free-standing birth centres in Germany

The history of free-standing birth centres in Germany provides context for understanding the settings in which the research was conducted. In many high-income countries, midwives can, in principle, care for women in all birth settings: in hospitals, free-standing birth centres, and at home. In reality, the scope of practice for midwives is often restricted either by policy or by supervisory authorities in each country's healthcare system (Galkova et al., 2022; ICM, 2017; Stone et al., 2023b). Historically, the professional scope of midwives across Europe, the USA, and Canada was restricted from the 19th century onward due to the growing influence of obstetrics and the formation of medical associations. Midwives, who were not allowed to obtain an academic education, became increasingly regulated and were relegated, especially in clinical settings, to the role of assistants to obstetricians (Metz-Becker, 2013). In Germany, as in other high-income countries, the majority of women gave birth at home until the 1950s (Schumann, 2009).[1]

In the 1980s, the first free-standing birth centres were established in Germany, the USA, and the UK (Ernst & Bauer, 2017; Stone, 2012; Walsh & Downe, 2004). These early birth centres were inspired by second-wave feminism and the demand by women for autonomy over their bodies and their medical care, including decisions about how and where to give birth (Stone, 2012). The term "being delivered" resonated with many second-wave feminists as emblematic of a loss of agency in childbirth. Rather than actively "giving birth," women often felt overly managed and positioned as passive recipients of medical interventions (Davis-Floyd, 1992; Hunter, 2006). The free-standing birth centre model foregrounds an organisational ethos in which care is centred on relationships with clients rather than on organising care around institutional flow. In contrast to free-standing birth centres, Walsh (2006, p. 1330) characterises hospital-based maternity care as resembling an "assembly-line," where care tends to be structured by an institutional rationality foregrounding control, surveillance, and the efficient management of bodies and time (Simonds, 2002).

The establishment of free-standing birth centres not only offered women an alternative choice to hospital birth, but also gave midwives the opportunity to practice their profession more fully, work independently, and offer one-to-one care to women seeking a low-intervention, physiological, or, in the terms of the 1980s, natural birth (Annandale, 1988; Davis-Floyd, 2018). While national guidelines exist for the operation of free-standing birth centres in Germany, their internal bureaucratic and organisational structures vary significantly. A common aim across birth centres, however, is to ensure continuity of care through the presence of a known midwife or through the presence of a team with whom the woman has already built rapport, thereby fostering trust and relational care.

In 2010, while I was collecting data for my master's thesis, I met Hanne Beittel, the initiator of the first free-standing birth centre in Germany (Beittel, 2010). Beittel had been a labour and delivery nurse in several cities in the USA, as well as in Paris and Berlin. In spite of her nursing experience, she was unable to advocate for herself while in labour and suffered traumatic births during which she had to fight off hospital staff who were determined to administer a form of anaesthesia called twilight sleep. Twilight sleep had a slow entrance into obstetrics at the end of the 19th century, gaining popularity in the 20th century in, e.g., Germany and Britain (Taylor, 2023). The mixture of scopolamine and morphine was meant to offer relief from what was thought to be unbearable labour pain, along with the additional effect of erasing the woman's memory (Taylor, 2023). Considered an outgrowth of first-wave feminist demands for choice in childbirth, twilight sleep offered women the option to remain oblivious to the birth, rather than endure the unpredictable "whims" of the physician (Kuo, 2021, p. 59). While twilight sleep was embraced by some women as a form of liberation from the pain and unpredictability of birth, its very premise stands in stark contrast to the consciousness and agency that second-wave feminists later sought to reclaim in childbirth. In my own midwifery training at the end of the 1990s, one of my midwifery teachers often told stories of having to restrain women on the delivery bed before administering twilight sleep to prevent the uncontrollable flailing that the anaesthesia triggered.

Against this background, Beittel pursued studies in sociology in the late 1970s, focusing her research on the position of women as patients in obstetrics, examined through the lenses of power, domination, and violence. To better understand the countermovement to violence in obstetrics, she took part in natural birth workshops in the early 1980s with Sheila Kitzinger, Michel Odent, and Kitty Reid, eventually bringing Kitty Reid's birth centre manual from the USA to Germany, adapting it for the German healthcare system. After founding a self-help group in 1982 called "Birth Centre for a Self-Determined Birth," Beittel sought midwives who would work in the birth centre, an endeavour that took nearly five years. On February 25, 1987, the first baby was born in the Birth Centre at Klausnerplatz in Berlin. While Beittel was pleased with the results of her efforts and that of the organisation she founded, she did not believe that creating new structures for giving birth would be enough. She felt that lasting change could only happen when the potential for violence in each individual person was diminished. Her approach reflected a belief that structural reform must be accompanied by an inner ethical shift, without which cycles of domination and harm would persist.

Framing practice: Health insurance, law, and midwifery in Germany

While the historical emergence of free-standing birth centres highlights the social and feminist movements that shaped their development, midwifery care in each country is also shaped by the healthcare and legal systems in which they are embedded. These regulate the scope of practice and care delivery. Therefore, before turning to the study, I will situate midwifery within the broader structures that frame practice. The German healthcare system, founded in 1883 under Chancellor Otto von Bismarck, is among the oldest social insurance systems in the world (Schölkopf & Pressel, 2014). Built on the principle of solidarity, it pools risk by requiring contributions based on income rather than individual health status. Around 85% of the population is covered by statutory health insurance, with the remainder holding private insurance (Busse & Blümel, 2014). Contributions are shared between employees and employers, and dependents are automatically covered. Unlike the UK's National Health Service (NHS), which is financed through general taxation, the German system is primarily funded through insurance premiums, with coverage and professional regulations largely codified in the Social Code Book. Both statutory and private health insurance companies in Germany reimburse free-standing birth centres for operational expenses and for the regulated costs of births, whether they take place in free-standing birth centres or at home. Free-standing birth centres are run exclusively by independent midwives, and clinical leadership is legally required to be held by a midwife.

Midwifery has a special legal status in Germany. Paragraph 4 (§4) of the German Midwife Law (*Hebammengesetz*) defines birth assistance as a so-called reserved activity (*vorbehaltene Tätigkeit*). This means that, except in emergencies, only midwives are legally authorised to provide birth assistance. Physicians must ensure that a midwife is called to every birth and may not act as the primary birth attendant. Their role is limited to surgical interventions such as caesarean sections, vacuum extractions, or emergency care. This provision, rare in international comparison, secures midwives' autonomy in attending births at home and in free-standing birth centres. However, in hospitals, midwives still work within obstetric frameworks and may be limited in their authority and autonomy. This highlights how Germany's legal framework formally protects midwives' central role in childbirth and provides the backdrop for the *ASK a Midwife* study.

The *ASK a Midwife* study: Acquisition of skills and knowledge of midwives

To work safely in any birth setting, midwives must adapt their skills to the individual and medical needs of the women they care for, while also navigating the bureaucratic structures and staffing conditions of their workplace (Coddington et al., 2017; Cronie et al., 2012). In hospital settings, midwives are required to have a broad range of clinical competencies to care for women with complex medical needs and heightened risk during labour and birth, and often care for two or more labouring women at a time (Nilsson et al., 2019; O'Connell & Downe, 2009). In contrast, midwives working in free-standing birth centres and at home births provide woman-centred care to support physiological birth, while also possessing the skills to recognise when circumstances require a timely transfer to the hospital (Stone et al., 2023b). In free-standing birth centres in Germany, midwives provide continuous one-to-one care throughout labour, with a second midwife called in to assist in the final stage of labour or earlier, when necessary. A meta-ethnography on the skills and knowledge of midwives working in free-standing birth centres and at home births found that, when transitioning into practice in these settings, midwives needed to broaden their clinical reasoning, drawing more heavily on embodied knowledge and a care philosophy grounded in relationality and support for physiological birth (Stone et al., 2023b).

In most high-income countries, the majority of clinical, hands-on midwifery training takes place in hospitals. As a result, most midwives do not have practical experience attending births in free-standing birth centres or at home when they finish their studies. In Germany, midwifery students have a 12-week externship with independent midwives (Plappert et al., 2024), which may include a placement in a free-standing birth centre, with a home birth midwife, or with a midwife who provides only antenatal and postnatal care. However, placements in free-standing birth centres and with home birth midwives are limited, and not all students can be accommodated. In Germany, midwives are legally permitted to attend births in all settings upon certification, regardless of where they completed their practical training. While an externship in a free-standing birth centre or at home births may provide valuable experience, it is not a legal prerequisite for working in these settings. Notwithstanding where skills were first developed, adapting to the distinct ethos and practices of a free-standing birth centre can be facilitated through an orientation period, which formed the context in which this study was situated.

The *ASK a Midwife* study explored how newly qualified midwives became oriented to practice in a free-standing birth centre, drawing on their lived experience and the lived experience of experienced midwives working alongside them. Because the majority of the newly qualified midwives who participated in the study worked in free-standing birth centres that also provided care at home births, their orientation encompassed the distinct spatial and relational dimensions of attending births in women's homes, as well. The descriptive aim of the study was to identify the skills and knowledge newly qualified midwives needed to develop in their first year, and to explore, through focus groups with experienced birth centre teams, the strategies and orientation practices that were utilised to cultivate this development. The team discussions provided insight into how orientation was structured and how experienced midwives fostered learning within the context of everyday care.

Underpinned by hermeneutic phenomenology, the study also attended to the newly qualified midwives' lived experience and meaning-making in their *being-in-the-world* as midwives. Through this lens, orientation came to be understood as a process of becoming attuned to the relational and embodied dimensions of midwifery care. The aim was not to generate theory or produce generalisable findings, but to explore newly qualified midwives' experiences as they entered into the unfamiliar world of a free-standing birth centre, and to interpret the unfolding of meaning in their *being-with* women, families, and colleagues during orientation and early practice.[2]

In addition to contacting free-standing birth centres by post, two organisations helped me find participants for the study: Q.U.A.G. (Society for Out-of-Hospital Births) and the Network of Free-Standing Birth Centres. Recruited over 21 months, 15 newly qualified midwives participated and were interviewed three times in the first year of their orientation in a free-standing birth centre. The first interview was conducted in their first six weeks, while the second interview took place after they progressed to a new phase in their orientation. The third interview was conducted 9–12 months after beginning their orientation and was scheduled based on their own assessment of having reached a further stage of independence. In addition to this, focus group interviews were conducted with 13 free-standing birth centre teams. The focus groups comprised two to five experienced midwives who had experience working with newly qualified midwives during their orientation period. The focus group interviews were transcribed as one voice, since it was common for the midwives to finish each other's sentences and add details to shared stories. In addition to the interviews, the newly qualified midwives left a total of 123 voice messages throughout their orientation using the Signal app (Stone & Thomson, 2025). They often sent the messages directly after or one day after a moving, unsettling, or new experience. Most of the messages were about births they had observed and, later on in their orientation, births they led as the primary midwife. Lastly, I conducted five rapid ethnography sessions, comprising more than 70 hours of non-participant observation in four free-standing birth centres. This provided opportunities for spontaneous conversations with individual midwives in the teams in which the newly qualified midwives were working.

In hermeneutic phenomenology, one method of working with transcripts is to craft the lived experience of the participants into stories. Unlike methods that rely on verbatim texts, such as grounded theory, in hermeneutic phenomenology, interpretation is central, and multiple understandings of participants' accounts are possible (Crowther et al., 2017). The stories in this book were crafted into stories using participants' words, with occasional paraphrasing or re-ordering of sentences to create narrative flow. Contextual details were retained. Disfluencies such as repetitions were removed, while the midwives' language and phrasing were preserved. Written first in German and then translated into English, the process was cyclical and reflective, supported by discussions with both the newly qualified midwives and the experienced midwives while visiting the free-standing birth centres. Crowther (2017, p. 8) writes: *Each crafted story provid[es] glimpses of what is unconcealed beyond the semantic assemblage of words, enabling insights into the sense of phenomena to emerge.* Crafting stories allows meaning to become visible, offering stories that invite recognition and connection; the *phenomenological nod* that signals when lived experience has been authentically conveyed (Van Manen, 1990/2016).

In this book, I share lived experience stories of newly qualified midwives who were becoming oriented to free-standing birth centre and home birth care at a time that was historically marked by reconfigured relationships. Everyday assumptions about care, contact, and connection were deeply disrupted, making their transition from hospital-based clinical training to free-standing birth centre and home birth care that much more exceptional. My goal with each chapter is to move back and forth between the parts and the whole, illustrating the newly qualified midwives' path through orientation. While the study is underpinned by hermeneutic phenomenology, I have engaged with their stories using various analytic methods, philosophical frameworks, as well as Greek mythology to interpret their lived experience and those of the experienced midwives working alongside them. Each chapter reveals a unique aspect of their orientation and integration into their team.

As such, this book contributes to scholarship in three ways: first, by illuminating the lived experience of newly qualified midwives in settings where midwives hold full professional authority; second, by demonstrating how orientation practices shape professional identity and embodied knowledge; and third, by using hermeneutic phenomenological inquiry to reveal deeper levels of skill acquisition of midwives in out-of-hospital settings (Stone et al., 2023a, 2024). In German, *Geburtshaus* (English: 'birth house') is the standard term for a free-standing birth centre. The facilities that took part in this study were all free-standing birth centres, midwife-led institutions that are physically and administratively separate from hospitals. For clarity and to retain the flow of the text, I use the terms free-standing birth centre and birth centre interchangeably.

Notes

1 Since 1975, the percentage of babies born in free-standing birth centres and at home in Germany has remained between 1.3 and 2.0 % Schäfers, R. (2024). *Qualitätsbericht 2023: Ausserklinische Geburtshilfe in Deutschland*. Retrieved December 12, 2024 from https://www.quag.de/downloads/QUAG_Bericht2023.pdf.

2 Several papers related to the study have been published in peer review journals. These are: Stone, N. I., & Thomson, G. (2025). Exploring newly qualified midwives' lived experiences of out-of-hospital births through voice messaging and interviews. *Int J Qual Methods, 24*, 1–16. https://doi.org/10.1177/16094069251346849.
, Stone, N. I., Thomson, G., & Tegethoff, D. (2021). Ask a midwife: A qualitative study protocol. *Int J Qual Methods, 20*, 1–7. https://doi.org/10.1177/16094069211048383.
, Stone, N. I., Thomson, G., & Tegethoff, D. (2023a, Dec 27). 'Bringing forth' skills and knowledge of newly qualified midwives in free-standing birth centres: A hermeneutic phenomenological study. *J Adv Nurs, 80*(8), 3309–3322. https://doi.org/10.1111/jan.16029.
, Stone, N. I., Thomson, G., & Tegethoff, D. (2023b, Apr 8). Skills and knowledge of midwives at free-standing birth centres and home birth: A meta-ethnography. *Women Birth, 36*(5), e481–e494. https://doi.org/10.1016/j.wombi.2023.03.010.
, Stone, N. I., Thomson, G., & Tegethoff, D. (2024, Oct 2). Tailoring midwifery care to women's needs in early labour: The cultivation of relational care in free-standing birth centres. *Midwifery, 140*, 104202. https://doi.org/10.1016/j.midw.2024.104202.

References

Annandale, E. C. (1988). How midwives accomplish natural birth: Managing risk and balancing expectations. *Soc Probl, 35*(2), 95–110.

Busse, R., & Blümel, M. (2014). Germany: Health system review. *Health Syst Transit, 16*(2), 1–296.

Coddington, R., Catling, C., & Homer, C. S. (2017, Feb). From hospital to home: Australian midwives' experiences of transitioning into publicly-funded homebirth programs. *Women Birth, 30*(1), 70–76. https://doi.org/10.1016/j.wombi.2016.08.001

Cronie, D., Rijnders, M., & Buitendijk, S. (2012, Sep-Oct). Diversity in the scope and practice of hospital-based midwives in the Netherlands. *J Midwifery Womens Health, 57*(5), 469–475. https://doi.org/10.1111/j.1542-2011.2012.00164.x

Crowther, S., Ironside, P., Spence, D., & Smythe, L. (2017, May). Crafting stories in hermeneutic phenomenology research: A methodological device. *Qual Health Res, 27*(6), 826–835. https://doi.org/10.1177/1049732316656161

Davis-Floyd, R. (1992). *Birth as an American Rite of Passage*. University of California Press.

Davis-Floyd, R. (2018). *Ways of Knowing about Birth: Mothers, Midwives, Medicine, & Birth Activism*. Waveland Press, Inc.

Ernst, K., & Bauer, K. (2017). *Birth Centers in the United States*. American Association of Birth Centers.

Galkova, G., Bohm, P., Hon, Z., Herman, T., Doubrava, R., & Navratil, L. (2022). Comparison of frequency of home births in the member states of the EU between 2015 and 2019. *Glob Pediatr Health, 9*, 2333794X211070916. https://doi.org/10.1177/2333794X211070916

Hunter, L. P. (2006, Mar-Apr). Women give birth and pizzas are delivered: Language and western childbirth paradigms. *J Midwifery Womens Health, 51*(2), 119–124. https://doi.org/10.1016/j.jmwh.2005.11.009

ICM. (2017). *International Definition of the Midwife: Scope of Practice*. https://www.internationalmidwives.org/our-work/policy-and-practice/icm-definitions.html

Kuo, J. (2021). The sunset of twilight sleep. *Berkeley Sci J, 26*(1), 58–60. https://doi.org/10.5070/BS326157109

Metz-Becker, M. (2013). Hebammen und medizinische Geburtshilfe im 18./19. Jahrhundert. *die hochschule: Journal für wissenschaft und bildung, 1*, 33–42. https://www.hof.uni-halle.de/journal/texte/13_1/Metz-Becker.pdf

Nilsson, C., Olafsdottir, O. A., Lundgren, I., Berg, M., & Dellenborg, L. (2019, Dec). Midwives' care on a labour ward prior to the introduction of a midwifery model of care: A field of tension. *Int J Qual Stud Health Well-being, 14*(1), 1593037. https://doi.org/10.1080/17482631.2019.1593037

O'Connell, R., & Downe, S. (2009, Nov). A metasynthesis of midwives' experience of hospital practice in publicly funded settings: Compliance, resistance and authenticity. *Health (Lond), 13*(6), 589–609. https://doi.org/10.1177/1363459308341439

Plappert, C., Bauer, N., Dietze-Schwonberg, K., Grieship, M., Kluge-Bischoff, Zyriax, B.-C., & Striebich, S. (2024). Academic education of midwives in Germany (part 1): Requirements for bachelor of science programmes in midwifery education. Position paper of the midwifery science committee (AHW) in the DACH association for medical education (GMA). *GMS J Med Educ, 41*(3), 1–16. https://doi.org/10.3205/zma001688

Schäfers, R. (2024). *Qualitätsbericht 2023: Ausserklinische Geburtshilfe in Deutschland*. Retrieved December 12, 2024 from https://www.quag.de/downloads/QUAG_Bericht 2023.pdf

Schölkopf, M., & Pressel, H. (2014). *Das Gesundheitswesen im internationalen Vergleich: Gesundheitssystemvergleich und europäische Gesundheitspolitik* (2., aktualisierte und erweiterte Auflage ed.). Medizinisch Wissenschaftliche Verlagsgesellschaft.

Schumann, M. (2009). *Vom Dienst an Mutter und Kind zum Dienst nach Plan: Hebammen in der Bundesrepublik 1950–1975*. V&R Unipress.

Simonds, W. (2002). Watching the clock: Keeping time during pregnancy, birth, and postpartum experiences. *Soc Sci Med, 55*, 559–570. https://doi.org/10.1016/S0277-9536(01)00196-4

Stone, N. I. (2012, Oct). Making physiological birth possible: Birth at a free-standing birth centre in Berlin. *Midwifery, 28*(5), 568–575. https://doi.org/10.1016/j.midw.2012.04.005

Stone, N. I., & Thomson, G. (2025). Exploring newly qualified midwives' lived experiences of out-of-hospital births through voice messaging and interviews. *Int J Qual Methods, 24*, 1–16. https://doi.org/10.1177/16094069251346849

Stone, N. I., Thomson, G., & Tegethoff, D. (2021). Ask a midwife: A qualitative study protocol. *Int J Qual Methods, 20*, 1–7. https://doi.org/10.1177/16094069211048383

Stone, N. I., Thomson, G., & Tegethoff, D. (2023a, Dec 27). 'Bringing forth' skills and knowledge of newly qualified midwives in free-standing birth centres: A hermeneutic phenomenological study. *J Adv Nurs, 80*(8), 3309–3322. https://doi.org/10.1111/jan.16029

Stone, N. I., Thomson, G., & Tegethoff, D. (2023b, Apr 8). Skills and knowledge of midwives at free-standing birth centres and home birth: A meta-ethnography. *Women Birth, 36*(5), e481–e494. https://doi.org/10.1016/j.wombi.2023.03.010

Stone, N. I., Thomson, G., & Tegethoff, D. (2024, Oct 2). Tailoring midwifery care to women's needs in early labour: The cultivation of relational care in free-standing birth centres. *Midwifery, 140*, 104202. https://doi.org/10.1016/j.midw.2024.104202

Taylor, E. (2023, Dec 19). Hanna Rion and the weekly dispatch's twilight sleep crusade. *Med Humanit, 49*(4), 659–667. https://doi.org/10.1136/medhum-2022-012595

Van Manen, M. (1990/2016). *Researching Lived Experience: Human Science for an Action Sensitive Pedagogy* (Kindle ed.). Routledge.

Walsh, D. (2006, Mar). Subverting the assembly-line: Childbirth in a free-standing birth centre. *Soc Sci Med, 62*(6), 1330–1340. https://doi.org/10.1016/j.socscimed.2005.08.013

Walsh, D., & Downe, S. M. (2004). Outcomes of free-standing, midwife-led birth centres: A structured review. *Birth, 31*(3), 222–229.

2

SPARKS

Pathways into free-standing birth centre practice

Introduction

This chapter explores why the newly qualified midwives in this study chose to begin their professional lives in free-standing birth centres. Their decisions were rarely spontaneous; instead, many of them traced their motivations to formative experiences, often prior to or outside of formal midwifery education. During their studies, these motivations were frequently tested, particularly in clinical place-ments where neither woman-centred care nor physiological birth was common-place. This chapter traces how these tensions shaped their desire to work in settings that aligned more closely with their vision of midwifery and where they hoped to learn how to accompany birth differently. The stories presented here reveal how values are held and carried forward in the face of compromise.

Do we ever know the true beginning?

Have you ever wondered when your journey truly began? Do you remember the first whisper of an idea that set everything in motion? Tracing back to that spark reveals the quiet undercurrent of timing in our experiences and the small but dynamic choices that carried and continue to carry us forward, bringing us to a pivotal moment where everything that came before comes together, and we find ourselves in a well-defined new place. Before securing a first job as a midwife, whether in a hospital, a free-standing birth centre, or at home births, the decision to commit to a programme of study often requires effort and perseverance. Once immersed in training, every birth, interaction, and decision, no matter how small, contributes to shaping a developing professional identity and reveals professional and personal allegiances. This perspective underscores the idea that professional

DOI: 10.4324/9781003591306-2

pathways are often not predetermined; they are shaped through reflection and responsiveness to unfolding experiences. As events begin to shape midwifery students, they may deviate reluctantly from their intended direction, unclear about how to move forward.

A decision, like a path, does not simply appear fully formed before us. For the newly qualified midwives who participated in this study, their choice to work in a free-standing birth centre was shaped by personal experiences, professional encounters, and a sense of what kind of role they wanted to have at the births of the women in their care. As they navigated the landscape of their studies, some paths felt more aligned with their emerging professional identity and core values than others. Therefore, before we do a deep dive into the stories they told about orientation, let us first visit their sparks and experiences as students.

Shifting perspectives: Questioning what we believe to be true

Among the newly qualified midwives in this study, most chose to keep their decision to work in a free-standing birth centre after finishing their studies a secret from the midwives and doctors in their clinical placement, as well as from their teachers and professors. One reason for this is the prevailing criticism towards free-standing birth centres (Arabin et al., 2013; Drife, 2007; Rayment et al., 2020). I believe this largely originates from a lack of understanding about the work done there. Midwifery practice in these settings remains understudied, and misconceptions abound. International research has frequently explored organisational structures, attitudes of service users, perspectives of midwives working in birth centres, and the process of transferring women from free-standing birth centres to hospitals during labour or postpartum (Blix et al., 2014; Brocklehurst et al., 2011; David et al., 2006; Grigg et al., 2015). Nevertheless, descriptions of actual clinical practice and decision-making in free-standing birth centres are limited (Stone et al., 2023a, 2023b; Walsh, 2006). This leaves hospital-based obstetricians, midwives, and labour and delivery nurses uncertain about the clinical standards and safety measures in free-standing birth centres and home births, often leading them to view these settings as unregulated and potentially unsafe (Chervenak et al., 2013; Grünebaum et al., 2015). For professionals accustomed to clinical practice in hospitals, it is easy to imagine that the same alarming emergencies they encounter on a somewhat regular basis also occur in free-standing birth centres. I found myself in this mindset after nine years of clinical practice as a midwife in a small labour and delivery ward with 1,200 births per year, as did the team I worked in.

The hospital where I worked served as the designated transfer facility for the nearby free-standing birth centre, which profoundly shaped my conception of birth centres and home birth, in spite of having had a home birth with my son years before. As a result, my experiences were almost entirely limited to women transferred during labour, most of whom arrived exhausted and visibly distressed. None of these transfers were dire emergencies. However, the majority of transferred women requested an epidural for pain relief so that they could rest, something they were certain they would not need when choosing the birth centre. Many ultimately required an oxytocin drip to augment contractions, and a vacuum extraction to assist with the birth. In essence, they had booked the low-risk, low-intervention package and had received everything they did not bargain for. Because I only encountered free-standing birth centre clients under these circumstances, my perception of them became skewed. The women seemed to push themselves beyond their physical limits just to avoid hospital births, a decision I struggled to understand at the time. Since I loved the labour ward where I worked, it was difficult to grasp why they hadn't chosen to come to us in the first place.

Then, I won a new perspective.

During my master's programme in public health, I wanted to intern at the nearby free-standing birth centre. I approached the director, whom I had worked with a few times at the hospital during transfers, asking her if I could conduct a feasibility study for my master's thesis. She welcomed me, as did the five midwives who were working with her at the time. I entered with an open mind, determined to observe without bias. As it turned out, that wasn't very difficult since the reality was undeniable: their work was so fundamentally different from mine in the hospital that it felt like stepping into an entirely new world. What began as a feasibility study developed into an ethnographic project, culminating in my master's thesis, which described the distinctive practice of supporting physiological birth in a free-standing birth centre (Stone, 2012).

Newly qualified midwives: Starting with a foundation of fear

This postdoctoral study about newly qualified midwives builds on my earlier research. One of the findings of that research was that midwives trained almost exclusively in hospital settings had to actively "unlearn" the intervention-heavy protocols they had internalised so that they could support physiological births in the free-standing birth centre. This process of unlearning is also a phenomenon that midwives with post-qualification experience in hospital labour wards encounter when they get oriented to home birth care (Coddington et al., 2020). Furthermore, newly qualified midwives face additional challenges when commencing work post-qualification, since they often have fears surrounding birth and care at birth that do not get adequately addressed during their studies (Dahlen & Caplice, 2014; van der Putten, 2008). The midwifery teams I spoke with while collecting data for *Ask a Midwife* explained that newly qualified midwives are influenced negatively by their instructors' attitudes towards free-standing birth centres and home birth, in addition to acquiring a fear of birth in general during their training. This posturing fosters a climate of uncertainty and apprehension towards midwifery care in every setting. As a result, many newly qualified midwives receive both overt and covert messages discouraging them from pursuing careers in out-of-hospital settings, and some begin to question whether such a path is even viable. During my visits to free-standing birth centres across Germany, I found that many were struggling to recruit midwives, a reflection, in part, of this climate of fear and hesitation.

Early stirrings towards a professional path

Caroline, one of the newly qualified midwives I accompanied during her orientation, had previously completed an externship with a home birth midwife during her studies. We met in one of the birthing rooms at her birth centre for all her interviews. During our first meeting, we sat in a room decorated in rich, deep colours that added warmth and comfort to the space. It was simple, neat, and homelike. As we settled in, a newborn's cries suddenly broke through the quiet, penetrating the walls. For a brief moment, I felt myself pulled towards the cry before returning to Caroline's voice, which carried its own urgency. She began recounting how she had decided to become a midwife.

She told me that, from the age of 15, long before she began her midwifery studies, she had harboured a vision of birth that, for her, was not rooted in any prior life experience. In her imagination, she envisioned a woman labouring in water in a darkened room. Rather than just being an image in her head, she described it as a mood that filled her spirit. She leaned into this feeling, seeking out everything she could find about birth. She was somewhat certain, even before her midwifery studies began, that she did not want to work in a hospital after qualifying. However, she sensed that sharing this openly would be controversial. She recalled how teachers actively discouraged students from considering this path after graduation. The story she tells below highlights how midwifery students develop a tacit awareness of which career paths are socially and professionally acceptable. Caroline told me:

> One of my externships was with a home birth midwife. I was on the road with her, so to speak, for two months and observed eight home births. She was a workaholic. It was exhausting AND incredibly beautiful. The way she worked matched exactly what I'd always imagined midwifery to be. It perfectly aligned with my expectations and was exactly what I'd envisioned. To me, home birth was just normal birth. That's how it should be. In my clinical placements, I always thought: "Gosh, what are you doing here? This is completely wrong—everything you're doing here is wrong. It just doesn't make sense." From day one, from the very first day in the clinic, I thought, "Oh God, what on earth are you all doing here?" So, yes, it was always the other way around. I never experienced clinical work—hospital obstetrics—as normal. I don't know where I picked that up; it was simply my gut feeling from the very beginning.
>
> I never shared this with anybody except for a few, select people. I was very aware that this was a sensitive topic. Um—I didn't just go around saying "What are you doing here? That's not right. I'll never work in a hospital." I mean,

I'm not stupid. I wanted to get through my clinical placements as best I could. I wanted to feel comfortable and get along with everyone. I'm good at adapting. I've always been like this. I got along fine outwardly, but inwardly I was always thinking, "Wow, are you all insane?!"

(Caroline, first interview)

Some midwives, like Caroline, speak of midwifery as a calling, sensing an alignment with the profession that often emerges well before formal training (Foley, 2004). These kinds of narratives influence how student midwives experience, and perhaps reject, aspects of midwifery training in hospitals, since they believe that birth is a physiological process best supported through presence, patience, and trust rather than intervention. This tension between inner conviction and institutional labour ward experiences echoes themes identified in other midwifery research on how dominant medical paradigms can conflict with more embodied ways of knowing and holistic understandings of birth (Davis-Floyd, 1994; Simonds et al., 2007).

Caroline's silence concerning her negative assessment of the medicalised births she witnessed in her clinical training was not unique among the study participants. Like her, Nina also struggled with the disconnect between her clinical practice and her deeper sense of how she wanted to practice midwifery. During her externship with an independent midwife, she gained insight into three different birth settings, experiences that reshaped her understanding of midwifery and birth.

Doing my clinical training in a hospital was a huge adjustment phase—the biggest one in my life. I knew that I wanted to work in a birth centre when I finished, but I let myself be influenced by what I was told in my training hospital. My clinical practice was in a Level 1 hospital with over 2,000 births—with breech deliveries and twins. Everyone said that, after passing my exams, I had to start in a hospital with high-risk births to be a good midwife. That idea stuck with me. Then I had an externship with an absolutely wonderful midwife who attended home births, birth centre births, and hospital births as an independent midwife. I spent six weeks with her, living in her home with her family, accompanying her in her work. It was a complete 'aha' moment. Even though I struggled at times—because I was deep in this phase of figuring things out and didn't know what to do, where to go, and everything felt so uncertain—that experience made one thing clear: there was no other path for me. I couldn't imagine working in a hospital. So, I started searching and ended up here.

(Nina, first interview)

Nina's experience of an adjustment period while getting oriented to and learning client care was common among all study participants during their midwifery studies. However, adapting to *how* things were done and accepting those practices were two different processes. For many midwifery students, the care they observe and are expected to provide in hospital settings during clinical training

often conflicts with their ideals of midwifery, as well as with the theoretical principles of the midwifery philosophy of care they have been taught (Bradshaw et al.,
2018; Ebert et al., 2016; Green & Baird, 2009; Schoene et al., 2023). This tension
is not unique to students; experienced midwives also report struggling to reconcile their desire to offer woman-centred care with the reality of hospital labour
wards (Lewis et al., 2020). Institutional structures often contribute to fragmented
models of care, whereby midwives are expected to simultaneously care for multiple labouring women, respond to phone calls, assess women as they arrive, and
manage administrative tasks. Under these conditions, which are shaped by staffing
shortages and a lack of continuity, students are required to adapt to a model of care
that prioritises institutional flow over the individual needs of labouring women
(Ebert et al., 2016).

In some cases, this disconnect does more than create dissonance; it becomes
a source of moral distress or even trauma. Some researchers have referred to this
experience as moral injury (Dean et al., 2019; Kendall-Tackett & Beck, 2022).
This is the psychological harm that arises when individuals are compelled to violate
their deeply held moral beliefs by acting against them. For student midwives, this
injury may emerge not only from what they are asked to do, but from what they
are unable to prevent and involuntary witness (Davies & Coldridge, 2015). Several
participants described feeling overwhelmed, disempowered, or ethically compromised by the care they observed and were expected to provide. Sally, a newly
qualified midwife, shared this with me:

> I didn't tell my teachers that I was starting at a birth centre because I was afraid
> that they would say: "You can't work **there** after your training." Birth centres
> and home births are really demonised. Even now, the people I worked with in
> my clinical trainings are probably thinking, "How stupid is that, seriously?"
>
> And it shouldn't be that way because I'm so proud to be where I am now and
> not in a clinic where I would constantly be worried about EVERYTHING. That
> fear and anxiety—I realise now—was there up until I finished my first month
> here at the birth centre. The anxiety had lingered on from school. A friend of
> mine during my midwifery studies actually quit in her third year. We had similar
> experiences, fears about being in the labour ward, wondering what would hap-
> pen today. Who will the patient be? Will the birth be awful? Traumatic? In the
> birth centre, it's different. We get excited when a woman calls in labour. The
> baby is coming!
>
> I was often really anxious during my clinical practice training. Why? Was
> that really necessary? Part of it is because of this horrible hospital hierarchy. As
> a student, you're expected to go along with everything all the time and not speak
> up. You may not want to. You might have different ideas in your head about how
> things should be done. And then you arrive, and they stomp you straight into the
> ground. And then, okay, you have to fight your way back up and get through it.
>
> *(Sally, first interview)*

In a survey of midwifery students in Germany, Schoene et al. (2023) found that nearly two-thirds (65.3%) had witnessed midwives performing interventions without the woman's consent during clinical placements, and more than half (51.8%) had observed midwives providing care that they interpreted as physical violence against labouring women. Reports were even higher for physicians, with three-quarters of students witnessing both non-consensual interventions (74.7%) and physical violence (74.3%). These experiences had a profound emotional impact: 91.9% of students who participated in the study reported symptoms associated with acute stress or PTSD. These findings are consistent with research by Fontein-Kuipers et al. (2016), which revealed that midwives' strong intentions to provide woman-centred care often clashed with institutional barriers, including time constraints, social norms, and a lack of supportive leadership. When ideals of care are continually compromised, students may begin to question the care they feel forced to provide, as well as their calling to the profession.

Research on disrespect and abuse during childbirth, though often situated in low-resource contexts, offers a broader framework for understanding how institutional conditions can undermine both providers and women. Ishola et al. (2017), for example, outline how structural factors such as staff shortages, overcrowding, and lack of privacy can lead to neglect or verbal abuse, whether intentional or not. Bohren et al. (2015) similarly show that mistreatment during childbirth can take many forms: overt acts like physical abuse, subtle forms such as neglect, or systemic failures that compromise dignity and privacy. Regardless of how they arise, these experiences can affect a woman's health, her experience of giving birth, and her right to receive respectful, humane care. Without time or space to process what they see, students may feel emotionally unmoored and isolated, unsure how to integrate their values into the practice they are being trained to deliver. For some, these moments leave lasting impressions of birth and what it means to be a midwife.

Staying the course

Yet rather than abandoning their training, the newly qualified midwives in this study remained committed to their ultimate midwifery goals, navigating environments that often conflicted with their emerging sense of what midwifery should be. Green et al. (2009) discovered in their UK study investigating attrition and retention of student midwives that

> students spent a long time trying to 'fit in' with clinical practice. There were accounts that if they spent too long questioning issues, it was easy to become labelled as 'a difficult student', instead it was about keeping 'quiet' and being accepted as part of the team.
>
> *(p. 84)*

As we saw in the interview narratives thus far, Caroline described adaptation as a strategy for perseverance, while Sally appeared to suppress her frustration, sensing it instead as anxiety. Nina, however, let her internal compass guide her towards care practices that made sense to her and aligned with her values. Her intention grew from acknowledging her gut feelings and allowing them to shape her path forward.

Not all of the newly qualified midwives in this study had negative experiences during their clinical training. Sheila, for example, spoke consistently with enthusiasm about the hospital where she trained. She felt that the way labouring women were cared for there aligned with how she envisioned her own future midwifery practice, and she hoped to work there after passing her exams. However, she noticed a significant drop in her stress levels during an externship at a free-standing birth centre, which reset her course. She said:

> During my training, I found that working in the hospital was actually quite nice and something I completely enjoyed. I liked the action, the adrenaline, and the complexity of special cases like twin births, high-risk pregnancies, and preterm births. Initially, I planned to stay in the hospital for a while to gain more experience. Then I did my externship at a birth centre. Over those five weeks, I noticed how my stress level dropped day by day. By the end, it was clear to me that this was where I wanted to work after finishing my training. Now, it feels like a second home to me.
>
> *(Sheila, first interview)*

What connects the stories of all the newly qualified midwives in this study is that their journeys were profoundly affected by their experiences in their clinical placements, as well as in their externships. Their growth, both professionally and personally, was shaped by the presence and ethos of others.

Some career paths initially seem clear and straightforward but may lead to unforeseen challenges or require re-evaluation, while others emerge unexpectedly, offering new opportunities through experience and adaptation. Not all paths lead to a predetermined destination. The journey for these midwives into free-standing birth centre practice was a process shaped by moments of uncertainty, reflection, adaptation, and courage.

Questions for reflection

1 Can you recall a moment before or in your early midwifery journey when something "clicked" or made sense in a new way?
2 What kinds of interactions or experiences spark a deeper sense of connection or purpose for you in your work?
3 How do moments of resonance or inspiration shape your understanding of what it means to be a midwife?
4 Write down the positive births you have experienced. What do these have in common?

References

Arabin, B., Chervenak, F. A., & McCullough, L. B. (2013, Feb). Die geplante Hausgeburt in industrialisierten Landern: Burokratische Traumvorstellung vs. professionelle Verant-wortlichkeit [Planned non-hospital births in industrialized countries: Bureaucratic dream vs. professional responsibility]. *Z Geburtshilfe Neonatol, 217*(1), 7–13. https://doi.org/10.1055/s-0032-1333215 (Die geplante Hausgeburt in industrialisierten Landern: Burokratische Traumvorstellung vs. professionelle Verantwortlichkeit.)

Blix, E., Kumle, M., Kjaergaard, H., Oian, P., & Lindgren, H. E. (2014, May 29). Transfer to hospital in planned home births: A systematic review. *BMC Pregnancy Childbirth, 14*, 179. https://doi.org/10.1186/1471-2393-14-179

Bohren, M. A., Vogel, J. P., Hunter, E. C., Lutsiv, O., Makh, S., Souza, J. P., Aguiar, C., Coneglian, F. S., Diniz, A. L. A., Tunçalp, Ö., Javadi, D., Oladapo, O. T., Khosla, R., Hindin, M. J., & Gülmezoglu, A. M. (2015). The mistreatment of women during child-birth in health facilities globally: A mixed-methods systematic review. *PLoS One, 12*(6), 1–32. https://doi.org/10.1371/journal.pmed.1001847

Bradshaw, C., Murphy Tighe, S., & Doody, O. (2018, Sep). Midwifery students' experi-ences of their clinical internship: A qualitative descriptive study. *Nurse Educ Today, 68*, 213–217. https://doi.org/10.1016/j.nedt.2018.06.019

Brocklehurst, P., Hardy, P., Hollowell, J., Linsell, L., Macfarlane, A., McCourt, C., Marlow, N., Miller, A., Newburn, M., Petrou, S., Puddicombe, D., Redshaw, M., Rowe, R., Sandall, J., Silverton, L., & Stewart, M. (2011, Nov 23). Perinatal and maternal outcomes by planned place of birth for healthy women with low risk pregnancies: The birthplace in England national prospective cohort study. *BMJ, 343*, d7400. https://doi.org/10.1136/bmj.d7400

Chervenak, F. A., McCullough, L. B., Grunebaum, A., Arabin, B., Levene, M. I., & Brent, R. L. (2013, Fall). Planned home birth in the United States and professional-ism: A critical assessment. *J Clin Ethics, 24*(3), 184–191. https://www.ncbi.nlm.nih.gov/pubmed/24282845

Coddington, R., Catling, C., & Homer, C. (2020, Sep). Seeing birth in a new light: The trans-formational effect of exposure to homebirth for hospital-based midwives. *Midwifery, 88*, 102755. https://doi.org/10.1016/j.midw.2020.102755

Dahlen, H. G., & Caplice, S. (2014, Dec). What do midwives fear? *Women Birth, 27*(4), 266–270. https://doi.org/10.1016/j.wombi.2014.06.008

David, M., Pachaly, J., Wiemer, A., & Gross, M. M. (2006, Oct). [Out-of-hospital births in Germany--a comparison of "large", "medium", and "small" free-standing birth cen-tres]. *Z Geburtsh Neonatol, 210*(5), 166–172. https://doi.org/10.1055/s-2006-951740 (Ausserklinische Geburtshilfe in Deutschland--Perinataldaten "grosser", "mittlerer" und "kleiner" Geburtshauser im Vergleich.)

Davies, S., & Coldridge, L. (2015, Sep). 'No Man's Land': An exploration of the traumatic experiences of student midwives in practice. *Midwifery, 31*(9), 858–864. https://doi.org/10.1016/j.midw.2015.05.001

Davis-Floyd, R. (1994). The technocratic body: American childbirth as cultural expression. *Soc Sci Med, 38*(8), 1125–1140.

Dean, W., Talbot, S., & Dean, A. (2019, Sep). Reframing clinician distress: Moral injury not burnout. *Fed Pract, 36*(9), 400–402. https://www.ncbi.nlm.nih.gov/pubmed/31571807

Drife, J. (2007). Do we have enough evidence to judge midwife led maternity units safe? No. *BMJ, Sep 29*(7621), 643. https://doi.org/10.1136/bmj.39343.461146.AD

Ebert, L., Tierney, O., & Jones, D. (2016, Jan). Learning to be a midwife in the clinical envi-ronment; tasks, clinical practicum hours or midwifery relationships. *Nurse Educ Pract, 16*(1), 294–297. https://doi.org/10.1016/j.nepr.2015.08.003

Foley, L. (2004). How I became a midwife: Identity, biographical work, and legitimation in midwives' work narratives. In M. T. Segal, V. Demos, & J. J. Kronenfeld (Eds.), *Gender Perspectives on Reproduction and Sexuality* (pp. 87–128). Elsevier.

Fontein-Kuipers, Y., Boele, A., & Stuij, C. (2016). Midwives' perceptions of influences on their behaviour of woman-centered care: A qualitative study. *Front Women's Health, 1*(2), 20–26. https://doi.org/10.15761/FWH.1000107

Green, S., & Baird, K. (2009, Feb). An exploratory, comparative study investigating attrition and retention of student midwives. *Midwifery, 25*(1), 79–87. https://doi.org/10.1016/j.midw.2007.09.002

Grigg, C. P., Tracy, S. K., Tracy, M., Schmied, V., & Monk, A. (2015, Sep). Transfer from primary maternity unit to tertiary hospital in New Zealand - timing, frequency, reasons, urgency and outcomes: Part of the evaluating maternity units study. *Midwifery, 31*(9), 879–887. https://doi.org/10.1016/j.midw.2015.04.018

Grünebaum, A., McCullough, L. B., Brent, R. L., Arabin, B., Levene, M. I., & Chervenak, F. A. (2015, Mar). Perinatal risks of planned home births in the United States. *Am J Obstet Gynecol, 212*(3), 350, e351–356. https://doi.org/10.1016/j.ajog.2014.10.021

Ishola, F., Owolabi, O., & Filippi, V. (2017). Disrespect and abuse of women during childbirth in Nigeria: A systematic review. *PLoS One, 12*(3), e0174084. https://doi.org/10.1371/journal.pone.0174084

Kendall-Tackett, K., & Beck, C. T. (2022). Secondary traumatic stress and moral injury in maternity care providers: A narrative and exploratory review. *Front Glob Womens Health, 3*, 835811. https://doi.org/10.3389/fgwh.2022.835811

Lewis, L., Barnes, C., Roberts, L., McLeod, L., Elliott, A., & Hauck, Y. L. (2020, Jul). The practice reality of ward based midwifery care: An exploration of aspirations and restrictions. *Women Birth, 33*(4), 352–359. https://doi.org/10.1016/j.wombi.2019.08.010

Rayment, J., McCourt, C., Scanlon, M., Culley, L., Spiby, H., Bishop, S., & de Lima, L. A. (2020). An analysis of media reporting on the closure of freestanding midwifery units in England. *Women Birth, 33*(1), e79–e87. https://doi.org/10.1016/j.wombi.2018.12.012

Schoene, B. E. F., Oblasser, C., Stoll, K., & Gross, M. M. (2023, Apr). Midwifery students witnessing violence during labour and birth and their attitudes towards supporting normal labour: A cross-sectional survey. *Midwifery, 119*, 103626. https://doi.org/10.1016/j.midw.2023.103626

Simonds, W., Rothman, B. K., & Norman, B. M. (2007). *Laboring on: Birth in Transition in the United States*. Routledge. Table of contents only https://www.loc.gov/catdir/toc/ecip075/2006028290.html

Stone, N. I. (2012, Oct). Making physiological birth possible: Birth at a free-standing birth centre in Berlin. *Midwifery, 28*(5), 568–575. https://doi.org/10.1016/j.midw.2012.04.005

Stone, N. I., Thomson, G., & Tegethoff, D. (2023a, Dec 27). 'Bringing forth' skills and knowledge of newly qualified midwives in free-standing birth centres: A hermeneutic phenomenological study. *J Adv Nurs, 80*(8), 3309–3322. https://doi.org/10.1111/jan.16029

Stone, N. I., Thomson, G., & Tegethoff, D. (2023b, Apr 8). Skills and knowledge of midwives at free-standing birth centres and home birth: A meta-ethnography. *Women Birth, 36*(5), e481–e494. https://doi.org/10.1016/j.wombi.2023.03.010

van der Putten, D. (2008). The lived experience of newly qualified midwives: A qualitative study. *Br J Midwifery, 16*(6), 348–358. https://doi.org/10.12968/bjom.2008.16.6.29592

Walsh, D. (2006). 'Nesting' and 'matrescence' as distinctive features of a free-standing birth centre in the UK. *Midwifery, 22*(3), 228–239. https://doi.org/10.1016/j.midw.2005.09.005

3

"I STILL FELT LIKE A STUDENT AT FIRST." STORIES OF BEGINNINGS

Introduction

Chapter 2 examined the underlying motivations that led newly qualified midwives to begin their careers in free-standing birth centres, often in quiet opposition to the norms encountered during their training. These decisions reflected personal conviction and a desire to enact a form of care that aligned more closely with their vision of midwifery. This chapter shifts the focus to what followed: the realities of beginning practice. It explores the complex process of transitioning from student to midwife, a shift that takes time and effort. Despite formal certification, many midwives described feeling hesitant, uncertain, and at times, as though they were stepping back into the role of student. These accounts reveal the emotional and professional dissonance that can accompany early practice and highlight how mentorship shaped their capacity to grow into the role.

The experience of early career midwifery

In general, when entering into professional midwifery practice, the transition into a new work environment requires both clinical competency and the willingness to broaden and deepen skills. Newly qualified midwives often feel challenged during the process of adapting to professional autonomy, with the dual responsibility of navigating a new clinical setting while keeping pace with expectations for their skill development. The first year can be a stressful period marked by anxiety, increased accountability, and significant adjustment to clinical responsibilities (Foster & Ashwin, 2014; Pairman et al., 2016). Structured transition programmes have been introduced internationally to address these challenges, offering support through mentorship and ongoing professional education

DOI: 10.4324/9781003591306-3

(Nolan et al., 2022; Pairman et al., 2016). Effective mentorship and preceptorship programmes provide invaluable guidance and professional support, which help new midwives develop confidence and competence (Foster & Ashwin, 2014; Wissemann et al., 2022). Furthermore, these supportive relationships foster a sense of belonging within the professional community, positively influencing career satisfaction and long-term retention in the midwifery workforce (Wissemann et al., 2022). Effective support during this transition is essential, and both mentorship and preceptorship play key roles in shaping a midwife's early career experience.

Mentorship differs from preceptorship and onboarding in several fundamental ways. Preceptors often take on the role of a supervisor and predominantly support a new colleague in their development of clinical skills. In preceptor relationships, supervision is often geared towards surveillance of skill acquisition, with regular assessments to ensure that milestones are being reached. With onboarding, a form of brief orientation, new colleagues learn what their duties are and where to access resources they might need. Mentorship, however, is geared towards helping a new colleague develop skills, as well as to achieve career success through overcoming challenges in their field. While mentorship shares some similarities with preceptorship, it differs in that it goes beyond supervision and assessment, emphasising a deeper, trust-based relationship where mentors and mentees take time to understand each other personally and professionally, something that is often less emphasised in preceptorship. The origins of mentorship can be traced back to ancient literature, where mentors were often depicted as essential to personal growth and success.

Athena and her role in the journey of Telemachus

When searching for examples of mentorship in mythology and history, the story most often referenced is that of Athena and Telemachus in Homer's *Odyssey* (2020), which is widely regarded as the first recorded account of a mentor–mentee relationship. Composed in the 8th-century BCE, the *Odyssey* tells of Odysseus's long journey home after the Trojan War. In his absence, his wife Penelope and their son Telemachus struggled to hold their household together under pressure from unruly suitors who overran their home. Athena, the goddess of wisdom, handicraft, and warfare, visited Telemachus disguised as Mentes, a trusted friend of Odysseus, whose name is the root of the word mentor. At a moment when Telemachus felt powerless, Athena encouraged him to begin his search for his father. She continued to guide him throughout his journey, sometimes in disguise, sometimes more directly, offering wisdom, protection, and reassurance when he felt unable to go on. Through this mentorship, Telemachus grew in confidence. Athena's guidance, though not always visible, shaped his development from an insecure youth into a capable leader.

Colley (2002) highlights how mentorship has historically been embedded within existing power structures, often reinforcing hierarchical relationships rather than fostering collective empowerment. This dynamic is also reflected in mythological narratives, where female mentorship is often absent or depicted as reinforcing male-dominated hierarchies, as in the story of Athena and Telemachus (Colley, 2002). Mythology and literature frequently depict women as rivals rather than allies, often positioning them in competition for power, status, or the favour of men (Lewis, 2011). Lewis (2011) noted that in the 1970s and 1980s, there was a movement to reconceive and rewrite fairy tales and myths to show women in a more positive light. Because the narratives that had been passed down reflected broader socio-cultural patterns in which women's power was limited and their alliances discouraged, retelling myths became an act of resistance, since historical representations of mentorship often focus on men guiding other men.

Good mentorship

As was evidenced by the relationship between Athena and Telemachus, mentorship is an evolving relationship in which a more skilled and knowledgeable individual serves as a guide, role model, educator, and advocate for someone with less experience. In midwifery, the mentor is meant to offer encouragement, discuss difficult situations, explore ways to grow in the professional field, and support the mentee to become a fully integrated professional in their field (Bradford et al., 2022). Forming a collegial friendship also belongs to good mentoring, in addition to a more modern view that mentorship should minimise power differentials that might arise due to the dissimilarity in professional experience (Johnson & Ridley, 2008).

Midwifery has long been rooted in shared knowledge and mutual support, going back to the time when the path to becoming a midwife was through apprenticeship training. While most midwives today practice in hospitals with unyielding hierarchical structures, mentorship could alleviate this by emphasising trust, reciprocity, and solidarity rather than perpetuating competition and conformity. In the free-standing birth centres where this research took place, the midwifery teams took collective responsibility for mentoring the newly qualified midwives. Some of the newly qualified midwives who worked in large teams (10+ midwives) had one or two designated colleagues whom they met with regularly, while in smaller teams, each experienced midwife took responsibility for the orientation and training of the new colleague. In several of the free-standing birth centres, the expectation that newly qualified midwives would observe and work alongside each colleague before practising independently gave each individual in the team a chance to build trust, while also gaining a clear sense of the new midwife's skills and approach to care.

Interviewing experienced midwifery teams gave me the opportunity to hear first-hand how they mentor and support new colleagues and gave me insight into how newly qualified midwives are integrated into the team. While newly qualified midwives are trained to gradually take on responsibility, their work never becomes fully separate from the work of their colleagues. In these settings, care is understood as a shared, team endeavour, and midwifery practice is built on collaboration and mutual support. One team described this process as follows:

Pam: There is generally one colleague who takes on the responsibility of mentor. She doesn't do everything, though. It's more that she, together with the new colleague, looks around to see who in the team can best answer a particular question. For example, I might tell my mentee: "Justine made this transition two years ago. Maybe ask her where she got additional funding." We try to make the entire team's knowledge available, including advice on how to manage finances better. The idea is to give them a strong start, so they don't fall into a financial hole and can, for example, pay for their insurance.

Ruth: Right. And we've also always integrated the new midwives during their orientation into the on-call fees that women pay, so they are already included and compensated as part of the team, even when they're still mostly observing. Otherwise, it could be a problem, since the observation phase varies in length, depending on what the new colleague needs to learn.

Pam: It's really individual and depends on what the new midwife feels ready for. Also, a newly qualified midwife is usually paired first with a colleague who already has a few years of professional experience and absolutely not with another recently qualified midwife.

Elisabeth: Generally speaking, it's about two to four weeks of just observing, without taking over any responsibilities, mainly to really understand how we work here. Because you can't just explain it; it's like describing food; you have to experience it. Honestly, it can take up to a year to fully understand our structure. So, the first two to four weeks are just about getting oriented and starting to get into action.

(Team 5, focus group interview)

Mentorship in these settings was rarely about one assigned person solely passing on knowledge. Instead, it was distributed, relational, and adaptive, based on what each new midwife needed in order to develop their skills and increase their knowledge. While the structure of orientation provided direction, it was through everyday interactions and honest feedback that their confidence grew. One team shared how they experienced this shift in a newly qualified midwife:

Annamarie: I have the impression that the new colleagues who decide to come here are consciously choosing this way of working and are really open-minded. We have a thorough and supportive orientation, where they can ask lots of questions and observe for a long time, until they decide that they are ready to start taking on more responsibility. I feel that the new colleagues are fully engaged and really want to learn. For example, Betsy—she is totally committed and notices what needs to be done. She feels comfortable asking for help, is curious and reflective, even though she is sometimes too self-critical. But it's clear that she wants to work here.

Samantha: I feel good about working with Betsy. I can see how she interacts with the couples—she has a good instinct for what they need, what she can say, and what she shouldn't say. I feel relaxed working with her. I can hand things over to her without worrying because I know her level of competence.

Annamarie: I think Betsy is a really good example because at the beginning she was very unsure. She had a lot of doubts and questions which she was honest about. In the beginning, we weren't sure she'd stay because she didn't seem particularly resilient. But that completely changed. Now she's a really solid part of the team and much more confident with the couples.

(Team 7, focus group interview)

These stories reflect that mentorship in free-standing birth centres includes upholding the conditions for trust, reflection, and growth. The guidance offered by experienced midwives helps newly qualified colleagues settle into their roles gradually, without the pressure to work independently before they are ready. Still, even with strong support, the move from student to practicing midwife was not always seamless because the transition demanded more than clinical competence. It required a new orientation towards midwifery care during pregnancy, birth, and the postpartum period.

Making the leap from student to professional

Having passed their qualifying exams and eager to begin their first job as midwives, the newly qualified midwives felt ready to provide care as fully fledged midwives. However, the transition for most of the midwives was at times physically and emotionally demanding. As other studies have shown, it is not uncommon for newly qualified midwives to experience a gap between what they were taught and the realities of practice (Shi et al., 2023). This tension between academic preparation and clinical realities is often described as the theory-practice gap (Griffiths et al., 2019), a challenge widely recognised in midwifery and nursing education. In Kool et al.'s (2023) Dutch study on this transition, they found that many healthcare systems lack structured orientation programmes for newly qualified midwives, whether in hospitals or in community settings such as home birth and free-standing birth centres. Stakeholders in their Delphi study agreed that workplace-based support, including a proper introduction, clear role expectations, feedback, backup during shifts, and mentoring, is essential. Yet systemic and organisational barriers continue to limit how consistently this support is offered.

I felt like I was still a student: Transitioning to a new identity and role

In the initial weeks of their orientation in their free-standing birth centre, many of the newly qualified midwives were expected to spend time observing their colleagues. After years of preparation and the excitement of finally becoming midwives, being placed back into an observational role sometimes felt frustrating and anticlimactic. Although observation was interesting at times, it could also feel boring or passive, especially for those impatient to take on professional responsibilities. Despite feeling well-grounded in theoretical knowledge and basic practical skills, many of the newly qualified midwives recognised that they still lacked the full range of skills needed for working independently in a birth centre. Being asked to observe, without yet acting, often threw them back into a student-like position. Annabelle reported the following:

> It was actually crazy. It felt so sudden that I was no longer a student. I was a midwife. But I couldn't quite grasp it—that I had somehow suddenly moved up. I still felt like the midwife I was observing was the **real** midwife. She knew everything, and I was the student. I didn't immediately manage to shift into a new way of thinking about myself. When I observed her at antenatal appointments, I often thought: Oh, should I get up and fetch something for her? Or maybe I shouldn't because I'm no longer the student? So that was difficult for me—to just take on a purely observational role, as I'm someone who likes to do things and be involved. Finding that balance—listening attentively and absorbing information—was definitely interesting. I was so relieved to be mentored. I've heard from many friends who started in hospitals that they barely received any orientation.
>
> *(Annabelle, first interview)*

Annabelle was astonished at the breadth and depth of information that she was absorbing in her early weeks of orientation. While she spent the first two to three weeks just listening and watching her colleagues conduct antenatal appointments, some of the other newly qualified midwives that participated in the study were expected to carry out a part of the appointments. Theresa, a newly qualified midwife who was keen to overcome her feeling of being a beginner, said:

> My colleagues wanted me to do the antenatal appointments with them right after I started. During the consultations, I mostly sat and listened. When it came time to do the urinalysis, measure blood pressure, do the Leopold manoeuvres [uterine palpation], and listen to the fetal heart, I did that. What surprised me at the beginning was my intense uncertainty—not because I didn't know how to do things or didn't trust myself, but because I did my clinical practice in a level one hospital that had what I would call a traditional training environment—we

always had to show someone what we were doing and get their approval. At the first antenatal care appointment I went to here at the birth centre, I didn't yet know the midwife I was shadowing and felt like the 'new one.' I questioned if she thought it was okay if I did something. I didn't dare just do the urinalysis and discard it afterwards. Of course, I'm a midwife now. I can assess things, and I know that I have the competence. But I didn't want to do anything without first asking my colleague. Totally ridiculous, actually. But at that moment, I felt uncertain.

(Theresa, first interview)

Theresa's account illustrates the uncertainty that newly qualified midwives can experience during their transition into their new work environment. Even though she felt confident in her abilities, she hesitated to act independently because her previous training environment had conditioned her to seek approval before carrying out clinical tasks.

Beyond simply acquiring new skills in their free-standing birth centres, the newly qualified midwives had to undergo a process of cognitive and emotional realignment, particularly in relation to their past experiences in hospital settings. They talked about how their mentors helped them to overcome the difficult and sometimes traumatic experiences they had had in their clinical training. Many described needing to reconcile or reframe the challenging and sometimes distressing events they had witnessed and participated in. This theme surfaced repeatedly in their narratives, reflecting the impact of prior institutional environments on their professional identity formation. Amelia, a newly qualified midwife who had experienced distress in her clinical placement during her studies, shared the compassion with which her mentor addressed her discomfort during a client's transfer from the birth centre to a hospital.

We had to transfer a woman during labour to the hospital. My colleague wanted me to go with, since I hadn't seen a transfer yet. I felt kind of sick to my stomach and must have sighed quite loudly because my colleague asked me if I had a "hospital trauma." I was so relieved that she said it out loud. I looked at her and said: YES--and then I was okay. There seems to be a consensus that midwifery students have really uncomfortable and intense experiences in their training in hospital labour wards. She didn't take my experience for granted. She knew how I felt and that reassured me. The best part was that, when we got to the hospital, everyone there was so nice. My colleague introduced me and said I was in my orientation. The midwife at the hospital took note of my name and spoke to me directly. It was a really good experience.

(Amelia, first interview)

These moments of acknowledgment and reassurance helped midwives like Amelia begin to rebuild their confidence after difficult experiences during their midwifery studies. Alongside emotional support, gradually taking on responsibilities was equally important in fostering a sense of readiness.

Throughout their orientation, each midwife progressed from observation to providing independent care. At Sheila's birth centre, readiness was not determined solely by the number of births that were attended, but also by how well the newly qualified midwife was integrated into the team. Sheila worked with each member of the team, observing how each one worked. In turn, she was observed by all of her colleagues as she gradually took on more responsibility during appointments. She said:

> So, I basically have two midwives in the team who mentor me and kind of also take care of me. I talk with both of them on a regular basis. We had agreed that I would first off observe each midwife during three to four antenatal appointments –and then conduct each type of appointment at least once with another midwife present. And then, gradually, I would transition to conducting appointments on my own. That's the stage I had reached, and then I just briefly checked in with my colleague, one of my mentor midwives, and she said: 'Yeah, all good. You can do it. Just make sure someone else is in the birth centre, and then it's fine.'

> *(Sheila, first interview)*

With time and support from their colleagues, the newly qualified midwives gradually built the foundation they needed to feel stable in their new roles. Theresa explained that the flat hierarchy at her free-standing birth centre helped her move relatively quickly from feeling like a student to feeling like a midwife. She was still less experienced than her colleagues, but fully integrated into the team. She believed that this early sense of belonging was central to her confidence and to her continued development of practical skills. Sheila similarly felt that being trusted by all of her colleagues to take on responsibility bolstered her confidence. Looking back on their early weeks and months, all of the newly qualified midwives expressed gratitude that their transition had been gradual.

The newly qualified midwives' experiences highlight the transformative power of mentorship when it is rooted in genuine encouragement and shared growth, rather than surveillance or rigid evaluation. Mentorship in midwifery should not only focus on skill acquisition, for it has the potential to be far richer than this, offering newly qualified midwives opportunities to find their footing and grow into their professional identities. In these spaces of collective support, it is possible for newly qualified midwives to shape who they want to become.

Questions for reflection

1 Think back to a time when you felt "like a student" even though you had stepped into a new professional role. What helped you begin to see yourself differently?

2 How have mentors or colleagues shaped your early professional identity? How do you support others who are not as far along as you are?

3 In what ways can collective mentorship (shared by a team) be more effective than one-to-one mentoring? What challenges might it bring?

4 When have you been supported to take on responsibility gradually (as opposed to quickly), and how did this affect your skill-building and confidence?

References

Bradford, H., Hines, H. F., Labko, Y., Peasley, A., Valentin-Welch, M., & Breedlove, G. (2022, Jan). Midwives mentoring midwives: A review of the evidence and best practice recommendations. *J Midwifery Womens Health, 67*(1), 21–30. https://doi.org/10.1111/jmwh.13285

Colley, H. (2002). A 'rough guide' to the history of mentoring from a marxist feminist perspective. *J Educ Teach, 28*(3), 257–273. https://doi.org/10.1080/0260747022000021403

Foster, J., & Ashwin, C. (2014). Newly qualified midwives' experiences of preceptorship: a qualiftative study. *MIDIRS Midwifery Digest, 24*(2), 151–157.

Griffiths, M., Fenwick, J., Carter, A. G., Sidebotham, M., & Gamble, J. (2019, Nov). Midwives transition to practice: Expectations and experiences. *Nurse Educ Pract, 41*, 102641. https://doi.org/10.1016/j.nepr.2019.102641

Homer. (2020). *The Odyssey* (E. R. Wilson, Trans.). W. W. Norton & Company.

Johnson, W. B., & Ridley, C. R. (2008). *The Elements of Mentoring* (Kindle ed.). St. Martin's Press.

Kool, E., Schellevis, F. G., Jaarsma, D., & Feijen-de Jong, E. I. (2023, Dec). How to improve newly qualified midwives' transition-into-practice. A Delphi study. *Sex Reprod Healthc, 38*, 100921. https://doi.org/10.1016/j.srhc.2023.100921

Lewis, S. (2011). Women and myth. In K. Dowden & N. Livingstone (Eds.), *A Companion to Greek Mythology* (pp. 443–458). https://doi.org/10.1002/9781444396942

Nolan, S., Baird, K., & McInnes, R. J. (2022, Nov). What strategies facilitate & support the successful transition of newly qualified midwives into practice: An integrative literature review. *Nurse Educ Today, 118*, 105497. https://doi.org/10.1016/j.nedt.2022.105497

Pairman, S., Dixon, L., Tumilty, E., Gray, E., Campbell, N., Calvert, S., Lennox, S., & Kensington, M. (2016). The Midwifery First Year of Practice programme: supporting New Zealand midwifery graduates in their transition to practice. *New Zealand College of Midwives Journal*(52), 12–19. https://doi.org/10.12784/nzcomjnl52.2016.2.12-19

Shi, J., Li, X., Li, Y., Liu, Y., Li, J., Zhang, R., & Jiang, H. (2023). Experiences of newly qualified midwives during their transition to practice: A systematic review of qualitative research. *Front Med (Lausanne), 10*, 1242490. https://doi.org/10.3389/fmed.2023.1242490

Wissemann, K., Bloxsome, D., De Leo, A., & Bayes, S. (2022, Jan-Dec). What are the benefits and challenges of mentoring in midwifery? An integrative review. *Womens Health (Lond), 18*, 17455057221110141. https://doi.org/10.1177/17455057221110141

4

BECOMING A PART OF BIRTH STORIES

Attuning to the whole

Introduction

In Chapter 3, we observed that most of the newly qualified midwives were impatient during the initial weeks of their orientation period, eager to begin independent practice in their free-standing birth centres. However, the experienced midwives required that newly qualified midwives first observe established practices before taking on responsibility, especially at births. In this chapter, we explore how newly qualified midwives, through observation and participation, began to get adjusted to the new setting. They became familiarised with routines through focused observation and documenting births, where they learned to pick up on subtle cues in shared practice.

How do we see the whole?

While the newly qualified midwives were well-prepared for hospital-based care and confident in meeting established clinical standards, care in free-standing birth centres is organised around the individual, whereby the goal is to understand the needs of the client within the broader context of her life. This was new to all of the newly qualified midwives. It necessitated a comprehensive understanding of the continuum of care that is offered in free-standing birth centres, spanning from early pregnancy through childbirth and into the postpartum period. This encompassed clinical procedures, as well as learning about and experiencing the emotional and psychosocial dimensions in each phase. Their midwifery education had provided a solid technical and theoretical foundation; however, the integrative knowledge required to support women over time was missing. Orientation became a kind of re-education, a way to come to know what holistic, comprehensive care feels like in practice. In Gadamer's (2004) terms, it required a shift in horizon.

DOI: 10.4324/9781003591306-4

Hans-Georg Gadamer (2004), a hermeneutic phenomenologist, uses the term horizon to describe the range of vision that frames what we can understand from a given position. He wrote that: *Horizon is not a rigid boundary but something that moves with one and invites one to advance further* (p. 238). With this image, Gadamer offers a way of understanding knowledge as something that shifts in relation to our experience and our environment. As Spence (2005) has written, Gadamer's concept of the fusion of horizons involves the way individuals' understandings may evolve and broaden through reflective engagement with the perspectives of others.

The horizon of the newly qualified midwives, shaped by their education and clinical experience in hospital settings, came into contact with another horizon: the care practised by experienced midwives, grounded in continuity, and marked by sustained familiarity with clients' medical and psychosocial histories. Orientation, in this sense, brought pregnancy care into view as an evolving, responsive practice centred in the life of each woman. Each phase: pregnancy, labour and birth, and the postpartum period carried its own significance and required its own form of care and attention, with care situated within the context of each person's life in response to their histories and unfolding needs across time. Importantly, the whole was not defined by birth as its endpoint. Care commonly continued into the postpartum period, making it possible to understand how pregnancy and birth influenced postpartum developments.

This view of care contrasts with prevailing models in modern healthcare, where repetition and specialisation are often equated with quality (Birkmeyer et al., 2002). For complex technical procedures such as cardiac surgery, centralising care in high-volume centres has been shown to improve outcomes. However, applying this logic to pregnancy and childbirth represents a category error. Birth, for example, is best understood as a physiological process rather than a pathological one (Renfrew et al., 2014; WHO, 2018). Treating it solely as a medical procedure risks unnecessary interventions and undermines the relational, woman-centred care essential to supporting physiological birth (Stone et al., 2023). In conventional quality management thinking, "process" is often equated with rigid standardisation: following the same steps in the same way for every case is understood as the best way to minimise variability and reduce risk (Donabedian, 1966/2005). However, in childbirth, and particularly in midwifery care, processes must remain flexible, relational, and responsive to the individual needs of each woman.

In midwifery education programmes, standardisation often takes the form of meeting numerical requirements for "catches" or deliveries, irrespective of time spent in actual care of labouring women. A Swedish study found that newly qualified midwives felt unprepared to offer appropriate support during labour, despite achieving the expected number of births (Schytt & Waldenström, 2013). In other words, no matter how many catches a student midwife or midwife has, numerical accumulation of births alone cannot equip her for the demands of practice in a free-standing birth centre, where the heart of care lies in relational and embodied dynamics, cultivated through listening, observing, and interacting, and which are fundamental to supporting physiological birth. Care is dynamic and requires developing sensitivity to labour rhythms, choosing interventions in the moment they become necessary (Miller et al., 2016). In addition to this, supporting physiological birth requires knowledge that is grounded in careful observation, patience, and trust in the labouring woman's competence. Midwives therefore need to be skilled in reading the subtle rhythms of birth, fostering connection, and creating an environment where labour can unfold without unnecessary interference, in addition to their clinical skills.

How to be a beginner: Being present without standing out

So, how do experienced midwives in free-standing birth centres help newly qualified midwives learn to care with appropriate responsiveness? One way is through requiring an observation period. In one of the focus groups, several experienced midwives reflected on the importance of beginning with observation. Observation is often seen as a passive act, however, at births in free-standing birth centres, it is a fundamental component of care. Learning to listen attentively, to wait, and to respond only after understanding the woman's needs in that particular situation was described as the essence of midwifery. Orientation was about learning to be present in a non-assertive, unobtrusive way and knowing why that matters. This perspective was echoed in the following focus group interviews.

Audrey: I think what makes this process of settling in so difficult is that it involves a kind of transition. But I also think it's an organic one.

Dana: I think it's really important that they start with observation because that is the essence of caring for women here at the birth centre: observing. What is the woman telling me? What does she need? And then waiting. It's not my role as a midwife to present myself and take over, but to take things in—to listen, to wait, to observe. That's why I think it's so important that a midwife is able to do this. And the orientation period is exactly the right time to show that you can learn this and eventually work this way.

(Team 1, focus group interview)

The expectation that midwives cultivate a quiet, attentive presence is not new. Historical midwifery texts often paired technical skill with particular attention to bearing, presence, and restraint (Sharp, 1985; Siegemundin, 1690/1992). Midwives were expected to carry themselves with humility and vigilance. Writing in 1671, Sharp (1985) warned midwives against premature intervention and urged close attention to the woman's own timing. For example, they should not rupture the membranes prematurely, nor should the birth be accelerated or forced, something she described as akin to torture. For Sharp and Siegemundin, intervening too soon, especially unnecessarily, risked serious harm. These were practical warnings, as well as being reflections of a worldview in which the timing of birth was governed by divine order. Learning to be present without dominating the space is a long-standing cornerstone of midwifery wisdom that has been neglected and forgotten in busy, institutionalised birth settings.

Because midwifery care in free-standing birth centres and at home is often equated with historical traditions of birth attendance, this form of care is sometimes dismissed as antiquated, even when it reflects evidence-based, relational practice. However, these early texts must be read in the context of their time. Figures like Sharp and Siegemundin wrote before the Enlightenment, in an era when medicine had not yet been transformed into a science that viewed bodies as discrete, mechanical systems. In their 17th-century writings, birth was portrayed as a natural process embedded in a divine order. A midwife's skill lay in anatomical knowledge together with knowing when not to act based on their trust that God would lead them, just as the labouring woman would be brought forth safely (or otherwise) according to a divine plan. These were not clinical judgements in the modern sense; they were matters of moral and theological interpretation, rooted in a worldview that is both conceptually and practically distant from the way care is understood and provided in today's free-standing birth centres. While the cosmologies that informed 17th-century midwifery have long since shifted, the practice of beginning with observation remains meaningful. No longer grounded in theological restraint, it now functions as a foundation for safe care, giving newly qualified midwives the opportunity to learn how care is shaped through responsiveness and presence. From that vantage point, they begin to understand how clinical judgement emerges from the integration of observation with research evidence and practice, and how this is applied within the context of each birth.

Hence, observation is a core component of clinical reasoning and judgement in free-standing birth centres. Yet, because it was not an emphasised part of the newly qualified midwives' clinical training, it can leave them feeling as though they are simply doing nothing in their first weeks and months of orientation. This tension between what observation offers and how it is experienced was a recurring theme in the focus groups. Team 7 discussed this:

Ashley: They often can't see how much they benefit from just observing us in the beginning. They start here after finishing their training and are highly motivated. They just want to get started. It's really difficult for them to wait so long. At first, they think it's great to just observe, but you can tell after two or three months that they want to be done with that. They want to be active and work on their own.

Heather: I think they feel as if we're holding them back—a little bit blocked, even. They would have liked to start sooner. And I often sense, especially with our new colleague, that this is creating some tension between us. I still remember something that the previous (newly qualified midwife) said at the end of her orientation when she began attending births on her own. She said: Now I understand how much that time helped me, now I understand why you structured it that way, and now I see what I got out of it. But for a long time, it was really difficult with her, as it is with (our current new colleague).

Nancy: I'm just wondering—how do they benefit from observation?

Francie: With the new colleague, I can see that she is in a position to just take in what's going on—to see how situations are handled. She's not yet in the role where she has to act or make decisions. Instead, she can absorb a lot, and maybe from that bit of distance, she can begin to see a fuller picture, to develop a sense of how things are done here, what options exist in specific situations, and how we might approach complex situations. And the more she observes and reflects, the more certain patterns begin to take shape. She has begun to understand how we respond in different situations, how decisions are made—not just clinically, but in relation to the woman and her needs. Over time, she has built a kind of working sense of what good care looks like here, and how to act in ways that are consistent with it.

(Team 7, focus group interview)

The experienced midwives who participated in the focus groups spoke about the challenges of orienting new colleagues, as well as what they look for, including what signals to them that a newly qualified midwife is beginning to understand what care means in the birth centre. One midwife reflected on a recent birth she attended with a new colleague:

Audrey: [I had a birth with a new midwife.] I reflected afterwards how it felt to work with her and really had the feeling that she knew what she was doing and why and asked questions when she wasn't sure. What I really liked about working with her was that she held herself back and observed what I was doing. She let me work. She didn't say much but still had a presence in the room. She was also very attentive. She listened to the fetal heart [with the handheld doppler]—she took responsibility for that—and was involved in what was going on without calling attention to herself. Our client remained the most important person in the room. Later on, during our client's active phase of labour, we worked more as a unit. The new midwife knew what I needed and was also paying attention to what our client needed. She noticed all the unspoken cues and was responsive. I found working with her really agreeable.

(Team 1, focus group interview)

This account illustrates that observation is not a placeholder for action but a deliberate, skilled form of care that is active, attuned, and grounded in responsiveness. It also shows that learning to offer care involves cultivating the ability to support labouring women through relational awareness and collaborative attention.

Documentation: Writing the birth story

Having considered what experienced midwives believe observation offers, what did the newly qualified midwives themselves come to understand and how? Documentation, in some free-standing birth centres, became a way of refining and initiating reflection, and in analysis, revealed itself as integral to the practice of observation. For Sally, a newly qualified midwife with a background in healthcare, this period of "just watching" became a form of discovery that revealed what her formal education had left out. She told me:

So, what and who am I watching? It's been different with each birth. Sometimes, I watch the midwife, like, her work, what she's doing and when. When is she listening to the fetal heartbeats? When is she doing a vaginal exam? How is she doing the vaginal exam? How does she "sense" what is happening when she is looking at or touching and palpating the outside of the woman's body? In other words, everything that I didn't necessarily learn in my training at the hospital. I feel like I need to observe those things. When is she talking with the other midwife (second midwife), what is she telling her, and how is she communicating with the woman? How is she communicating things with the woman, like transfer? How does she do that without creating fear? Choosing the right words seems super important.

And also, for example, the couples, how they are "being-with" each other. It's the couple relationship that I'm focusing on at the moment—just observing how they are with each other during labour because I totally missed that in my training. The partner was pretty much ignored. It's also really special to write that down and to listen exactly to how they interact with each other. For example, when I document births here, I write down a short summary: Martin gives Martina water and gently caresses the top of her head. Also, things like—he motivates her and says: "You can do it! We're a team." It really touches me deeply that the couples are so full of respect and love in this situation and that I can be there. It's also really special to write that down and to listen exactly to how they interact with each other. We also don't write anything like—head is cutting through. We write that the head is crowning. There's less violence in that. We didn't talk about this at all during my midwifery schooling. Not in classes and not at the hospital in the practical training. The hospital wanted it like this: Head is cutting through. There was a real emphasis on the documentation being as medical and as brief and concise as possible without any other part of the birth story. Here, we write in the partogramm the actual sentences that are spoken. It's sometimes so sweet because they don't know that they're going to get this story as a gift, and that they'll hear it again from the midwife. Their reactions are really special. They say: "Hey, wild! I said that?" They get totally emotional.

(Sally, first interview)

Sally's use of documentation to reflect on her profound realignment with the birth practices in her free-standing birth centre touched me deeply. In hermeneutic phenomenology, poetry can offer a way to engage more deeply with the stories that are shared. Green et al. (2021) write that poetic expression can help the researcher attend more closely to meaning as it emerges. I did not set out to write poetry during data analysis, however returning again and again to Sally's story led me to write a poem that expresses something that other interpretive analyses might have missed. This is the poem that I was inspired to write after reflecting on Sally's story:

A Crowning Achievement

I'm finding expressions of strength
To replace the violent ones I learned
From instructors who taught cutting words.
Women:
gently stroked,
Caught by waves unaware.
Rushing through and over,
Being sculpted
Not severed.
Connected
Through the expressions
I inscribe on indifferent paper,
Concealed between her screams and his affection
I am embedded in these birth stories for all time.
I choose to embolden,
Knowing her joy when she hears
What she has accomplished.

Just as Sally's reflections revealed how observation could open up new ways of seeing and documenting care, Nina's experience reveals how documenting births helped her to explore other avenues of perception. In her story, she recounts exploring what it feels like to listen to birth as opposed to seeing birth. For her, documenting birth connected her more profoundly with the birth process.

My first birth here—it was during the night—I was immediately, without question, the colleague. After I arrived (at the birth centre), I was immediately in the birthing room. I took off my shoes, went into the room, and whispered: "Hi." The primary midwife, who was listening to the fetal heart beats in that moment, asked me: "Can you write that down?" So, I simply started to document everything that I observed and became the storyteller.

Sometimes, I find it challenging to write down what the midwife said—like, do I write it down from a professional point of view or do I summarize the content? For example, I write the first sentence like this: The woman is now clearly vocalizing louder. And then I write: the name of the midwife, then a colon, and then underneath that I quote her: "There is so much space. Trust yourself." I write it like that because it is so beautiful to read what was said in each moment. I know in the back of my mind that we'll go over the birth documentation with the couple (several weeks) after the birth. When they hear their birth story, they say things like: "Wow! Really? I said that? Amazing!"

Most of the time at a birth, I'm watching the midwife. Simply watching what she's doing. And—different from the births that I saw in my clinical training (at hospital births), here I sometimes don't actually "see" anything, like when the head is born or the rest of the birth. Because, first off, it's not in my line of sight, and also because I've honestly seen that often enough. Besides, the three of them—the midwife, woman and her partner—are somehow in harmony with each other. So, I sit there with a bit of distance between myself and them and am only partially "in the bubble" with them. I'm observing. I don't get up and move if the woman moves from a kneeling position to the birthing stool—I don't move extra just to be able to see something better. I wouldn't do that because it would immediately attract the attention of the other three.

[At this birth, I realized]: Right! In my practical training, I was always the one who was standing or sitting in front of the woman and had a direct view. I could see that the head was emerging—or not. Here, I can't see it—I simply have to hear it… because I'm not yet the midwife who is at the perineum. So, now I have to somehow know differently what I can't see. I look at what the midwife is doing, or I hear a change in the woman.

(Nina, first interview)

This story captured a central theme of this chapter: how through documentation and observation, the shift from task-oriented care to seeing the whole took place. Nina's description illustrated how the process of documenting the birth could help her engage her senses, facilitating a new way of seeing and sensing birth. Her story also led me to work with poetic reflection as a way of engaging phenomenologically with the meaning that was taking shape.

The Storyteller

My first birth.
I entered the darkened room with a whisper,
Taking my place in the boat at the edge of rushing waves,
Careful not to disrupt the ebb and flow of gentle voices and
The roar of the lioness.
I knew I would document.
I didn't know I would be the storyteller.

The Storyteller:
Seemingly as old as time itself,
Honoured, valued in ancient societies,
Painted on cave walls,
What memory desired to nourish.
First pictures, then words, written in eternal ink,
A retainer of the past,
a form for the future,
a House of Being.
Now, in this birthing room,
I try to watch but am partially unsighted,
Unable to decipher and interpret with eyes and hands,
To see and feel the shock of hair,
Head crowning.
Now I listen for changes, screams, cries, voices,
Put pen to paper,
And compose a story for all eternity:
The beginning of a life.

In documenting births as a story, the newly qualified midwives developed their ability to observe relationships and interactions, integrating these into documentation that also preserved the forensic detail necessary for legal and clinical review.

The newly qualified midwives began their orientation with solid clinical skills and broad theoretical knowledge; however, care provision in the free-standing birth centres demanded a different set of skills. Beginning their orientation with observation was more than a pause before action. It was an invitation to experience a model of care that gave them opportunities to connect with the individuals in their care. In documenting births, they began to understand the significance of birth stories and their role as a midwife in them.

Questions for reflection

1 When you think back on your own learning so far, how has observation shaped the way you understand midwifery care? What have you learned through observing rather than doing?
2 In your training or practice, have you ever felt impatient during a period of observation? How might you reframe that time as an active form of learning rather than "doing nothing"?
3 Documentation in the birth centres was described as a way of deepening observation and reflection. How might your own style of documentation influence the way you perceive and remember care?

4 What do you notice when you begin to look beyond clinical tasks, such as watching how couples interact, or how the atmosphere in a room shifts? How might these observations shape your presence as a midwife?
5 Gadamer's concept of a "fusion of horizons" suggests that our understanding expands when we encounter new perspectives. In what ways have your horizons shifted through your experiences of practice so far?

References

Birkmeyer, J. D., Siewers, A. E., Finlayson, E. V., Stukel, T. A., Lucas, F. L., Batista, I., Welch, H. G., & Wennberg, D. E. (2002, Apr 11). Hospital volume and surgical mortality in the United States. *N Engl J Med, 346*(15), 1128–1137. https://doi.org/10.1056/NEJMsa012337

Donabedian, A. (1966/2005). Evaluating the quality of medical care. *Milbank Q, 83*(4), 691–729. https://doi.org/10.2307/3348969

Gadamer, H.- G. (2004). *Truth and Method* (J. Weinsheimer & D. G. Marshall, Trans.; 2nd rev. ed.). Continuum.

Green, E., Solomon, M., & Spence, D. (2021). Poem as/and palimpsest: Hermeneutic phenomenology and/as poetic inquiry. *Int J Qual Methods, 20*, 1–9. https://doi.org/10.1177/16094069211053094

Miller, S., Abalos, E., Chamillard, M., Ciapponi, A., Colaci, D., Comande, D., Diaz, V., Geller, S., Hanson, C., Langer, A., Manuelli, V., Millar, K., Morhason-Bello, I., Castro, C. P., Pileggi, V. N., Robinson, N., Skaer, M., Souza, J. P., Vogel, J. P., & Althabe, F. (2016, Oct 29). Beyond too little, too late and too much, too soon: A pathway towards evidence-based, respectful maternity care worldwide. *Lancet, 388*(10056), 2176–2192. https://doi.org/10.1016/S0140-6736(16)31472-6

Renfrew, M. J., McFadden, A., Bastos, M. H., Campbell, J., Channon, A. A., Cheung, N. F., Silva, D. R. A. D., Downe, S., Kennedy, H. P., Malata, A., McCormick, F., Wick, L., & Declercq, E. (2014). Midwifery and quality care: Findings from a new evidence-informed framework for maternal and newborn care. *Lancet, 384*, 1129–1145. https://doi.org/10.1016/S0140-6736(16)31472-6

Schytt, E., & Waldenstrom, U. (2013, Feb). How well does midwifery education prepare for clinical practice? Exploring the views of Swedish students, midwives and obstetricians. *Midwifery, 29*(2), 102–109. https://doi.org/10.1016/j.midw.2011.11.012

Sharp, J. (1985). *The Midwives Book*. Garland Pub.

Siegemundin, J. (1690/1992). *Die königliche Preußische und Chur-Brandenburgische Hoff-Wehe-Mutter, das ist: ein höchst nöthiger Unterricht von schweren und unrechtstehenden Geburthen* (Nachdruck ed.). Elwin Staude Verlag.

Spence, D. G. (2005, Sep). Hermeneutic notions augment cultural safety education. *J Nurs Educ, 44*(9), 409–414. https://doi.org/10.3928/01484834-20050901-05

Stone, N. I., Thomson, G., & Tegethoff, D. (2023, Apr 8). Skills and knowledge of midwives at free-standing birth centres and home birth: A meta-ethnography. *Women Birth, 36*(5), e481–e494. https://doi.org/10.1016/j.wombi.2023.03.010

WHO. (2018). *WHO Recommendations: Intrapartum Care for a Positive Childbirth Experience.* WHO recommendations, Issue.

5

OPENING UP PANDORA'S JAR

Honouring the power in women's stories

In Chapter 4, we saw how newly qualified midwives gradually learned to see the whole and began to grasp the broader rhythms of midwifery care in free-standing birth centres. For this process to occur, observation was a necessity. It was a way of engaging their senses and opening up to the relational and temporal whole of care. Their clinical education had prepared them to carry out tasks, but orientation demanded a shift in understanding care as situated, relational practice. In this chapter, the experiences of newly qualified midwives will be explored as they learn to support women through the physical and emotional landscapes of pregnancy. If observation marked the beginning of the newly qualified midwives' learning, then it was in antenatal care that they began to recognise how their presence could become part of the care itself. The presence they had been practicing started to take shape in how they listened, responded, and made space for trusting relationships.

The story of Pandora's jar

The myth of Pandora and her jar originates in ancient Greek mythology and can be found in the story of Prometheus and his brother Epimetheus (Buxton, 2004). According to Hesiod, Pandora was the first mortal woman, fashioned by Hephaestus at Zeus's command. Her name, Pandora, meaning "all gifted," is ironic since she was destined to bring chaos into the world. Though outwardly beautiful, she was intended as a divine punishment for humanity, specifically for Prometheus, who had defied Zeus by stealing fire and giving it to mortals.

Zeus instructed the gods and goddesses to give Pandora enchanting attributes, qualities that made her irresistibly alluring. As a final gift, the gods gave her a jar (sometimes referred to as a box in later retellings) with strict instructions not to open it. The jar contained all the evils of the world, including disease, suffering,

DOI: 10.4324/9781003591306-5

greed, and death. Despite the warning not to open the jar, Pandora's curiosity got the best of her. She opened it, flooding the world with all the evils that had been hidden inside. Although she put the lid back on as fast as she could, the only thing that remained in the jar was hope. This story is often interpreted as the origin of human suffering, with the remaining hope representing the possibility of redemption or solace in times of hardship.

Hope, as the last element remaining in Pandora's jar, suggests the enduring resilience of the human spirit even in the face of overwhelming challenges. Ernst Bloch (1986) wrote in his philosophy of the 'not-yet' that hope and longing never leave us. For Bloch, hope is interwoven in the present moment and, in this sense, serves as a bridge between the present and an imagined future, offering a sense of possibility and direction. In the context of pregnancy and birth, hope has the potential to be a guiding force, providing strength and direction.

Pregnancy as a conditional state

In Germany, pregnancy has been referred to as *in guter Hoffnung sein* since the 13th century, which translates to "to be in good hope" or idiomatically, "to be expecting." Historically, pregnancy has always been a time of uncertainty, and despite advances in antenatal care and medical technology, it remains so today. Sociologist Barbara Katz Rothman (1986/1993), in her book *The Tentative Pregnancy*, describes pregnancy as increasingly conditional due to the rise of prenatal examinations like amniocentesis. Amniocentesis is a diagnostic procedure in which a small sample of amniotic fluid is extracted from the uterus using a thin needle, typically guided by ultrasound, to test for genetic disorders and chromosomal abnormalities. Along with blood tests and ultrasound scans, such technologies have shifted pregnancy from an internal, embodied experience to an externalised medical process, where risk assessment and surveillance take precedence over conceptions of pregnancy as natural and normal (Stone et al., 2022). Rather than simply expecting a child, pregnant women now navigate a landscape of medical screenings, hoping for good test results and a fetus free from abnormalities (Erikson, 2007).

Because of this sense of tentativeness, many women choose not to announce their pregnancies until after the 12th week, or even later if they plan to undergo amniocentesis. The capability of advanced medical technology to offer a glimpse inside the womb has fostered both awe and apprehension, where uncertainty and wonder exist side by side. While seeing a growing fetus can feel miraculous, ultrasound technology is not designed to celebrate the wonder of life. Instead, as Erikson (2007) notes, sonographers conduct scans to identify potential anomalies, reinforcing pregnancy as a medicalised process rather than a natural one. Consequently, pregnant women are often described as future-oriented, constantly envisioning and taking the steps needed to ensure their unborn child's well-being and potential, even altering their behaviour and eating habits according to the latest recommendations (Lupton, 2012). Moreover, routine interactions with medical professionals are often described as one-sided, where healthcare professionals focus on gathering measurable, quantifiable data to confirm a diagnosis while sometimes dismissing clients' subjective experiences (Pilnick & Dingwall, 2011). In response to this medicalised experience of pregnancy, many women seek alternative models of care that prioritise a more holistic and personalised approach, such as giving birth in a free-standing birth centre or at home.

Being registered at a free-standing birth centre

At initial antenatal appointments in the free-standing birth centres participating in this study, the midwives reviewed their potential client's medical history to assess eligibility for birth at the birth centre. During these consultations, midwives discussed pregnancy-related concerns, individual and familial health, as well as emotional and psychological well-being. If none of the exclusion criteria were met, registration could proceed. In general, most free-standing birth centres require clients to attend at least four appointments during pregnancy with the midwifery team. While some women continue parallel care with their OB/GYN, others opt for exclusive midwifery care at their free-standing birth centre, as those admitted are typically considered at low risk for complications and do not need surveillance from a physician (Stone et al., 2022).

During these appointments, the midwives, pregnant women, and their families build a foundation for collaborative and relational care, since midwives do more than "just checking" during antenatal appointments (Skeide, 2019, p. 241). In the course of antenatal exams, midwives cultivate intimacy with their clients, in part through discussion, as well as through the Leopold manoeuvres (palpation of the woman's abdomen, uterus, and baby) (Stone et al., 2022). Engaging through dialogue and physical interaction also encourages a deeper level of contact between the woman and the midwife, the woman and her baby, and the midwife and the baby. These are building blocks for a collaborative, co-responsive relationship, whereby trust develops, strengthening the foundation for care (Peters et al., 2020). Midwifery care in free-standing birth centres thrives on engagement, responsiveness, and relational depth (Stone et al., 2024; Walsh, 2006).

Antenatal exams: Opening up Pandora's jar

When reflecting on their observations of antenatal exams, newly qualified midwives expressed astonishment at the depth of empathy and compassion demonstrated by their more experienced colleagues. During these appointments, they witnessed how their colleagues explored their clients' inner worlds with them; worlds shaped by personal histories, aspirations, and often unspoken traumas. Rather than simply delivering information, midwives engaged in dialogue, allowing women to voice their hopes and fears. This approach helped women to access and discover their own inner and outer resources, fostering agency and self-efficacy throughout pregnancy. Through this process, both midwives and their clients learned to navigate the complex physical and emotional terrain of pregnancy together. Over time, newly qualified midwives came to understand that their grounding presence helped guide women back to their inner strength during moments of uncertainty, helping prepare them for birth and parenthood.

Toni, a newly qualified midwife in a free-standing birth centre with 100+ births per year, described her beginning weeks of orientation as tedious and even boring at times. Like most of the newly qualified midwives, Toni wanted to jump into her new position and initially felt held back, in particular, by the time spent observing antenatal appointments. Many of the newly qualified midwives felt they had learned the basic components of antenatal exams during their theoretical studies, but they had not anticipated how much time midwives at the free-standing birth centre devoted to physical assessments and narrative engagement with the women. For several, measuring blood pressure, conducting a urinalysis, measuring the distance from the fundus to the symphysis, checking for oedema and varicose veins— in other words, solely checking physical parameters—was sufficient.

However, early on, newly qualified midwives observed that their experienced colleagues deliberately opened Pandora's jar, creating space for deeper emotions and concerns to surface as an integral part of care. Toni shared a story about this during her first interview, six weeks into her orientation.

When I leave work, I am often in awe of how amazing my job is. I love hearing how my colleagues guide women during appointments— how they've dealt with difficult topics, which words they've used, and how they've expressed issues. Sometimes I'm really surprised because I wouldn't have dealt with an issue the way they did. The midwives here are very open and will bring up everything that seems to be getting in the way of connecting. Sometimes, they discover that something distressing is buried deeply within our client, and they bring it out in the open. I remember an appointment where I was just observing. A couple came with their first child to an antenatal appointment because they couldn't organise a babysitter. Somehow, they got to talking about that child's birth, which had been borderline traumatic. I was fascinated at how the midwife discussed this experience with them, without pathologizing any part of it. She didn't discuss each moment with them. She let the couple talk about what was important to them. Occasionally she picked out an aspect of their story and said: How do you want to deal with this during this birth in case the situation is similar? I could see that it was having a very therapeutic effect. She used short anecdotes and storytelling from her own work as a midwife to open the door to possible solutions, without forcing a solution on them. I couldn't figure out in the beginning how she was choosing the stories, yet each and every story had the effect that the couple was able to see everything from a new perspective. The midwife had built such a profound connection to the couple. I had the feeling that she could see all the important issues as if they would be hanging in the air! She was able to pull them all out of thin air and address them, one after the other. After that appointment, I asked myself if I would ever be able to do that. A few weeks after that I had progressed in my orientation and was conducting antenatal exams alone. A woman came in who had stress at home and at work. I thought I was offering good solutions, but she rejected each one. I then just settled into listening to her and stopped trying to tell her how to solve her problems. After she finished telling me what was going on, I asked her simple questions: What needs to happen for you to feel better? Which part of this do you need help with? Which part can you do yourself? I suddenly had the feeling that I can do this because I created a protected, undisturbed space, like a bubble, for both of us. Even if the doorbell rings, and my next client is here, I know that I have enough time to listen to the client I'm with.

(Toni, first interview)

Toni first observed how her colleague gently uncovered a client's fears and unspoken emotions, and later, in her own interaction with a client, recognised how essential it was for her client to voice her experiences and navigate her own path. It was as if, by making space for these conversations, the midwives had opened Pandora's jar, wholly unafraid of the chaos they might unleash, ready to let something positive emerge. By listening deeply and holding space, they witnessed how meaning took shape and how hope surfaced in unexpected ways.

Issues that hang in the air

The neo-phenomenologist Hermann Schmitz offers a distinctive perspective on human experience by differentiating between the perception of individual elements in a situation or space and the holistic sensation of atmospheres or impressions (2011). Central to his philosophy is the concept of the *felt body* (*Leib*), which he distinguishes from the physical body (*Körper*). The physical body is the tangible, visible, and measurable body studied by the natural sciences and examined during antenatal care: it is the body as an object. The felt body, in contrast, encompasses the immediate, pre-reflective experiences and sensations that a person has of their own body. These are the sensations that occur that are perceived as tension, contraction, relaxation, or unease, before conscious thought. Schmitz argues that these involuntary bodily sensations form the basis of subjective experience. They are felt as an inner mood, both physical and emotional, before they have been fully reflected upon.

This distinction between the physical body and the felt body is particularly relevant in midwifery practice, where intuitive knowledge plays a significant role. Ólafsdóttir's (2009) research explores the relationships midwives forge with women during childbirth, arguing that through these connections, midwives cultivate an inner knowing, a deeply embodied form of knowledge. While often dismissed in formal training for lacking scientific grounding, this form of inner knowing, which includes intuition based on experience and pattern recognition (Benner, 1984), as well as intimate connections with women, has been shown to be valued by midwives (Crowther, 2020; Davis-Floyd & Davis, 1996). Ólafsdóttir's findings also highlight how the act of being-with women (*yfirseta*) fosters emotional connection, builds trust, and strengthens midwifery practice. She describes how midwives' stories reflect their experience of the atmosphere surrounding their clients. Hammond et al. (2013, 2014) maintain that midwives engage with birth spaces as lived, affective environments rather than birth being just a sequence of physiological events. The way midwives move within, adjust, and attune themselves to these spaces is a relational process, one that shapes the atmosphere of birth itself.

These ideas come into sharper focus when we examine Toni's story of her colleague's interaction with a client, where she felt as if there was something "hanging in the air." Schmitz explains that feelings are phenomena that are not limited by the boundaries of the body (2011). He ascertains that the felt body and the physical body are a whole entity, giving the example that sensing emotion is a physical experience. When someone is gripped by fear or brimming over with joy, it radiates outward and can be felt by others (Langewitz, 2022). In Schmitz's analysis, this takes the shape of an atmosphere that surrounds and connects people.

Toni had the feeling that there was something clearly present yet non-material and intangible around their client, something hanging in the air, that prompted the midwife she was observing to change her focus from the physical exam to a narrative interaction with her client. In both of Toni's stories, she first witnessed and then practiced what Dr. Rita Charon describes as eliciting narrative knowledge from a patient (2001). Providing time and space for a client to tell their story adds a dimension of personal meaning to a clinical interaction. Through listening to a story that moves the client or patient, the medical practitioner develops narrative competence and is also *moved*. Narrative competence, according to Charon, *is the competence that human beings use to absorb, interpret, and respond to stories. This… suggests that [narrative competence] enables the physician to practice with empathy, reflection, professionalism, and trustworthiness* (2001, p. 1897). Listening empathically to a client's story gives space for that client to tell their whole story, especially their fears and hopes.

Just as Toni recognised the presence of something intangible in her client's experience, Tara, whose story I will share next, also encountered a moment where listening became central to a woman's discovery of the hope that lay hidden underneath her previous, undisclosed fears.

Awakening hope: Tara's story

Tara was in the first month of her orientation as the holidays approached. At her birth centre, orientation was well-structured and defined through phases. Phase one, the phase that Tara was in, meant that she observed antenatal appointments as well as births. During phase one, her colleagues expected her to observe, without putting pressure on her to demonstrate competence or meet performance expectations. Tara enjoyed simply getting a feel for the rhythm of the antenatal appointments. She especially appreciated the depth of the interactions with clients and came with previous experience in a health-related field, which helped her connect almost effortlessly with a distressed client.

> There was a woman who came to us for an antenatal appointment just before we closed for Christmas and New Year's. She was in her 37th week of pregnancy and was glowing as she said: "Starting Saturday, I'm allowed to give birth here." The first day that women are allowed to give birth here or in any birth centre for that matter is 37 + 0 weeks [of pregnancy]. Well, she was sitting there and actually had to pause regularly to breathe through contractions. After a few of these contractions, she told us that she was planning on "keeping her baby inside" until Saturday so that she could give birth at the birth centre. My colleague looked at her and told her that we close for the holidays on Friday, December 24th, so she wouldn't be able to come on Saturday. Of course, the woman was devastated. She was sobbing. It was really awful for me to watch.
>
> I had read in her medical history that she had a traumatic birth in the hospital with her first child. She cried at her first appointment here when she talked about it. As I watched her, I could see that she had never really processed her trauma from the first birth. I have experience working with people with PTSD from my previous job. Between the traumatic birth of her first child and this pregnancy, she had a miscarriage—and a second bad experience at the hospital. She had been longing to give birth to this baby with us at the birth centre, and now she was hearing that she maybe wouldn't be able to come here. We were all really hoping that she was just having some sort of practice contractions or lightening and that they would eventually go away, but she was really having to breathe through them. It was hard to know for sure. It was a horrible situation.
>
> My colleague explained to her that she could call us on January 2nd—that we would be available for births after 9am, but, honestly, it really looked as if that wouldn't happen. She asked if she could at least see the birthing rooms again. My colleague said goodbye to her, and I went with her to this room where we are right now. She started opening up to me because I had said to her during her appointment that it would be good if she could find someone to talk about her first birth with. She had never done that, never gone for therapy, or gone back to the people who had been at her birth—the midwife and doctor—or even talked about it with anyone.
>
> So, we talked. I told her that I could tell that her first birth wasn't healed yet, and that it was bubbling up to the surface—sort of triggered by the contractions—as well as triggered by hearing from us that we would be closed for a week. I know that this can really get in the way of having a different experience with the next birth—a more positive experience. I gave her some suggestions—like

writing a letter and sending it to the hospital or even writing a letter and burning it. I told her that it would make sense to talk about it with someone, maybe not the actual midwife at the hospital—but, in general, to talk with a midwife or a therapist who had experience with this. And, if she couldn't find anyone to talk to, that writing a letter could really help to at least get clear about her feelings and make space for herself to have a different experience with this birth. Well, that was part one of the story. It isn't over yet. Here is the amazing part:

I told her: you know what, I have a feeling that you are going to come here on January 2nd and give birth to your baby. These contractions will probably go away. The baby is just getting settled—engaging with your pelvis. You have a chance now to work through some of the feelings that are left over from your first birth. I can't promise it, and maybe I shouldn't even say it, but I can really imagine you coming here on January 2nd. You had said that you wanted someone to photograph your birth. When you come, I'll still be in my orientation period as the third midwife, so I'll just be present at the birth observing. I can be your private photographer—as a special gift.

On January 2nd, I got a phone call in the morning from my colleague, who told me that this woman was at the birth centre with contractions. Her membranes had ruptured around 2am and her contractions started around 8am. When I arrived at the birth centre, she was leaning on her elbows on a table, breathing through a contraction. When it was over, I went over to her, and she fell into my arms. We both got so emotional, and then she said to me: You were right. I thought long and hard about what you said. After I left the birth centre that day, all my contractions stopped, and I didn't have another one until this morning.

She gave birth so beautifully here. I took so many photos, and, afterwards, she told me that it was the birth she had dreamed of. And really, it was so clear that everyone in the room felt a closeness—it was a really, really beautiful birth for all of us. I had so much joy for her in my heart—that she was so happy and had felt so good. I had so hoped that she would come, and that I would be at her birth. I felt so connected to her. It was beautiful.

(Tara, Interview 1)

By cultivating openness and dialogue, midwives facilitate a process whereby clients can make sense of their past experiences and envision new possibilities. Of course, it may not always lead to such an abrupt cessation of contractions, and no doctor or midwife can truly promise a client that working through previous, unresolved fears and trauma can pave the way for a desired outcome. However, research suggests that fear and anxiety during labour can significantly affect the birthing process. Adams et al. (2012) found that women with pronounced fear of childbirth experienced labour durations approximately 1 hour and 32 minutes longer than those without such fear. Even after adjusting for factors such as parity and medical interventions, the difference remained significant at 47 minutes. Similarly, Størksen et al. (2013) found that a previous subjectively negative birth experience increased the odds of developing fear of childbirth nearly fivefold, an association that was stronger than that between objective obstetric complications and subsequent fear. Therefore, when a woman's fear is alleviated in a stressful situation, it could have an effect on her physical body and, subsequently, on her labour.

Yet not all women who have experienced obstetric complications develop fear (Storksen et al., 2013), and some even look forward to future births despite previous difficulties. Rilby et al. (2012) found that women's feelings about future childbirth could range from dread to delight, shaped by their past experiences and also by the support they received from midwives, along with their desire to have more children. This underscores the complex emotional interplay surrounding childbirth, where fear, anxiety, and past trauma can coexist with hope, anticipation, and resilience. McKelvin et al. (2021) highlight that a woman's experience of childbirth is shaped by medical events, together with the emotional support she receives, her sense of control, and the opportunity to process past experiences. Their review suggests that fear, past trauma, and a lack of emotional support may contribute to distressing births, whereas midwifery-led relational care may foster feelings of security. In this way, narrative engagement becomes more than a communication tool; it is an active practice that supports women in reinterpreting their experiences and fostering a sense of agency. By creating an environment where past fears can be acknowledged and processed, midwives contribute to emotional well-being and to the physiological unfolding of labour itself (Crowther, 2020; Davis-Floyd & Davis, 1996).

Hope, trust, strength

Just as Pandora's jar held both suffering and hope, during pregnancy, uncertainty and possibility coexist. The medicalisation of pregnancy, while it contributes to feelings of tentativeness, has also provided invaluable tools that have saved lives. Narrative medicine, which, in straightforward terms, is simply listening to a client, does not mean turning away from these advances; rather, it calls for a recognition that knowledge is multi-faceted. In addition to clinical knowledge, relational and embodied knowledge has its place, since birth is not just a physical event: it is an experience shaped by human connection and presence. In moments of uncertainty and transition, receiving help can steady us and remind us of our strength when we begin to doubt ourselves. The newly qualified midwives learned to provide medical oversight while creating a relational space where fear can be expressed and confidence can emerge. In our most vulnerable moments, whether in pregnancy, labour, or life itself, building trusting relationships cultivates strength. Perhaps, as the first human woman, Pandora's hope was always hers to keep, no matter how long she kept the lid off the jar.

Questions for reflection

1 What do you think about Toni and Tara opening Pandora's jar?
2 How can you create space for hope in your practice?

3   What does it mean to you to balance and integrate medical knowledge with relational knowledge?

4   Have you ever experienced a moment where something was 'hanging in the air'? How did you respond?

References

Adams, S. S., Eberhard-Gran, M., & Eskild, A. (2012, Sep). Fear of childbirth and duration of labour: A study of 2206 women with intended vaginal delivery. *BJOG, 119*(10), 1238–1246. https://doi.org/10.1111/j.1471-0528.2012.03433.x

Benner, P. (1984). *From Novice to Expert, Excellence and Power in Clinical Nursing Practice*. Prentice Hall.

Bloch, E. (1986). *The Principle of Hope* (1st American ed.). MIT Press.

Buxton, R. G. A. (2004). *The Complete World of Greek Mythology*. Thames & Hudson.

Charon, R. (2001, Oct 17). The patient-physician relationship. Narrative medicine: A model for empathy, reflection, profession, and trust. *JAMA, 286*(15), 1897–1902. https://doi.org/10.1001/jama.286.15.1897

Crowther, S. (2020). *Joy at Birth: An Interpretive, Hermeneutic, Phenomenological Inquiry*. Routledge.

Davis-Floyd, R., & Davis, E. (1996, Jun). Intuition as authoritative knowledge in midwifery and homebirth. *Med Anthropol Q, 10*(2), 237–269. https://doi.org/10.1525/maq.1996.10.2.02a00080

Erikson, S. L. (2007, Dec). Fetal views: Histories and habits of looking at the fetus in Germany. *J Med Humanit, 28*(4), 187–212. https://doi.org/10.1007/s10912-007-9040-2

Hammond, A., Foureur, M., Homer, C. S., & Davis, D. (2013, Dec). Space, place and the midwife: Exploring the relationship between the birth environment, neurobiology and midwifery practice. *Women Birth, 26*(4), 277–281. https://doi.org/10.1016/j.wombi.2013.09.001

Hammond, A. D., Homer, C. E., & Foureur, M. (2014, Summer). Messages from space: An exploration of the relationship between hospital birth environments and midwifery practice. *HERD, 7*(4), 81–95. https://doi.org/10.1177/193758671400700407

Langewitz, W. A. (2022, Aug). The lived body (Der Leib) as a diagnostic and therapeutic instrument in general practice. *Wien Klin Wochenschr, 134*(15–16), 561–568. https://doi.org/10.1007/s00508-021-01911-1

Lupton, D. (2012). 'Precious cargo': foetal subjects, risk and reproductive citizenship. *Critical Public Health, 22*(3), 329–340. https://doi.org/DOI: 10.1080/09581596.2012.657612

McKelvin, G., Thomson, G., & Downe, S. (2021, Sep). The childbirth experience: A systematic review of predictors and outcomes. *Women Birth, 34*(5), 407–416. https://doi.org/10.1016/j.wombi.2020.09.021

Ólafsdóttir, Ó. Á. (2009). Inner knowing and emotions in the midwife-woman relationship. In B. Hunter & R. Deery (Eds.), *Emotions in Midwifery and Reproduction* (Kindle ed.). *11*, 3930–4280. Palgrave MacMillan.

Peters, M., Kolip, P., & Schafers, R. (2020, May). A theory of the aims and objectives of midwifery practice: A theory synthesis. *Midwifery, 84*, 102653. https://doi.org/10.1016/j.midw.2020.102653

Pilnick, A., & Dingwall, R. (2011, Apr). On the remarkable persistence of asymmetry in doctor/patient interaction: A critical review. *Soc Sci Med, 72*(8), 1374–1382. https://doi.org/10.1016/j.socscimed.2011.02.033

Rilby, L., Jansson, S., Lindblom, B., & Martensson, L. B. (2012, Mar-Apr). A qualitative study of women's feelings about future childbirth: Dread and delight. *J Midwifery Womens Health, 57*(2), 120–125. https://doi.org/10.1111/j.1542-2011.2011.00113.x

Rothman, B. K. (1986/1993). *The Tentative Pregnancy: Prenatal Diagnosis and the Future of Motherhood.* Norton Paperback.

Schmitz, H., Muellan, R. O., & Slaby, J. (2011). Emotions outside the box—The new phenomenology of feeling and corporeality. *Phenom Cogn Sci, 10*, 241–259. https://doi.org/10.1007/s11097-011-9195-1

Skeide, A. (2019, Jun). Enacting homebirth bodies: Midwifery techniques in Germany. *Cult Med Psychiatry, 43*(2), 236–255. https://doi.org/10.1007/s11013-018-9613-8

Stone, N. I., Downe, S., Dykes, F., & Rothman, B. K. (2022, Jan). "Putting the baby back in the body": The re-embodiment of pregnancy to enhance safety in a free-standing birth center. *Midwifery, 104*, 103172. https://doi.org/10.1016/j.midw.2021.103172

Stone, N. I., Thomson, G., & Tegethoff, D. (2024, Oct 2). Tailoring midwifery care to women's needs in early labour: The cultivation of relational care in free-standing birth centres. *Midwifery, 140*, 104202. https://doi.org/10.1016/j.midw.2024.104202

Størksen, H. T., Garthus-Niegel, S., Vangen, S., & Eberhard-Gran, M. (2013, Mar). The impact of previous birth experiences on maternal fear of childbirth. *Acta Obstet Gynecol Scand, 92*(3), 318–324. https://doi.org/10.1111/aogs.12072

Walsh, D. (2006). 'Nesting' and 'matrescence' as distinctive features of a free-standing birth centre in the UK. *Midwifery, 22*(3), 228–239. https://doi.org/10.1016/j.midw.2005.09.005

6

EMBODIED PRACTICES

Giving voice to lived experience

Introduction

In Chapter 5, we explored how the figure of Pandora, so often understood as a symbol of unleashed chaos, might instead be seen as an opening to presence and hope. In this chapter, we follow newly qualified midwives beginning to navigate what it means to be present with others as they develop their relational skills. Their skills and knowledge were cultivated through hands-on procedures such as the Leopold manoeuvres (abdominal palpation), as well as through observation and personal, shared, and embodied reflection.

Entering into mutual interaction

Individualised care implies an encounter. To care in the context of a free-standing birth centre is to take time to engage with clients in a way that allows them to be seen and heard. In this light, the myth of Echo, as rendered in Ovid's (2004) *Metamorphoses*, reveals a deeper phenomenological insight when agency and reciprocity are inhibited. Once an enchanting woodland nymph, Echo is punished by Juno and loses the ability to initiate speech; she can only repeat the last words spoken by others. After falling in love with Narcissus, she follows him through the forest, longing to reveal herself to him. She watches him, aching for contact and yearning for her love to be returned. However, when she finally meets him, she is only able to echo his words. She exists within the encounter silently, unable to shape it because she lacks the capacity to respond in her own voice. Incapable of letting go of her love for Narcissus, she wastes away in the forest, leaving behind only an echo.

What Echo's predicament reflects is a deeper phenomenological structure. What happens when we become invisible, and the conditions for agency and meaningful

DOI: 10.4324/9781003591306-6

exchange are denied? Although Echo is present with Narcissus, she cannot contribute meaningfully to the interaction. Her speech is controlled entirely by the language of the other. This dynamic offers a useful analogy for practitioner-client interactions, especially when technologically mediated care is relied on to the exclusion of a patient's or client's subjective, embodied experience. During pregnancy, obstetric ultrasound is used to determine gestational age, assess for fetal abnormalities and development of organs, and determine fetal position. The use of these technologies reconfigures the pregnant woman's body as a site of observation, translating her experiences into data that are intelligible to clinicians but don't necessarily reflect her experience (Lupton, 1994/2012), producing a clinical reality that may bypass her interpretive authority altogether (Stone et al., 2022). In this way, technology risks 'othering' the pregnant woman, reducing her to a monitored object within a system of care from which she is often relationally excluded. Even if she were to speak, she may not be heard. Care, when solely considered as a series of technologically mediated tasks, does not require the practitioner to have a personal interaction with a client or patient. Patients feel excluded from their own care, when what they need is interaction and confirmation (Drew, 1986).

The limits of measurement and the lived body

In the scientific worldview rooted in positivism, what is considered valid knowledge is grounded in observable, measurable indicators. Within this objectivist framework, the body is treated as separate from the person's inner life and subjective experience. Medical practitioners, who attend primarily to what can be measured, quantified, compared, and verified, seek distance, which is best achieved by minimising or eliminating subjectivity. Personal experiences and feelings, along with the meaning this has for the individual, are often downplayed, since subjectivity is seen to interfere with neutrality, reliability, and the pursuit of a diagnosis (Berg & Harterink, 2004).

This line of thinking is grounded in the work of René Descartes, the Enlightenment philosopher best known for the statement, "I think, therefore I am" (2007). His dualist philosophy separated mind and body, positioning the thinking mind as distinct from the physical body. Within this framework, the body is considered an object, something that can be fragmented, examined down to its smallest units (such as cell structures), researched, incised, altered, and acted upon through substances and chemicals. The mind and spirit are either dismissed altogether or treated as separate forces that influence the body, much like any other external force.

Challenging the objectivist tradition, phenomenological thinkers reconceptualised the body as lived, perceptual, and relational. Merleau-Ponty (1958), a French phenomenologist, sought to transcend the Cartesian separation of body and mind. For him, the body is not an object among other objects in the world; it is the very medium through which the world is encountered. He referred to this as the *lived* body (*le corps propre*), a term that emphasises the non-objectifiable, experiential body. This is the body that perceives, moves, and feels (Merleau-Ponty, 1958). As such, it is not the anatomical body of biomedical science; it is *my* body—the body I live—and does not require deliberate thought in order to function. For example, I do not need to reflect on my muscles and how they work in order to walk down the street. As Merleau-Ponty wrote: *It is never our objective body that we move, but our phenomenal body...* (1958, p. 121). He theorised that our phenomenal or sensing body, and not just the visible, physical body, is always oriented towards and engaged with the world.

An important precursor to these ideas can be found in the work of neuropsychologist Kurt Goldstein (1934), who postulated that illness is not simply a breakdown in one part of the body, but a disturbance in the organism's total relation to its environment. From this perspective, the body cannot be reduced to a set of mechanical parts and functions; it must be understood as a whole, unified field of sense, action, and orientation. Goldstein's work laid the foundation for later phenomenological accounts, such as Merleau-Ponty's, which rejected the notion of the body as a passive object in the world, viewing it instead as a sensing presence always situated within it.

Arriving at a deeper understanding of body

Further, the body is not a tool operated by a detached mental self; it is the lived medium through which we perceive, act, and experience meaning. People generally move through the world with a tacit awareness of their body until something changes, such as a broken leg, illness, stroke, or pregnancy, making the world suddenly seem foreign and more difficult to manoeuvre in. During pregnancy, physical changes can feel disruptive at times, influencing how women feel, respond physically, and navigate daily life. For example, certain smells may become suddenly intolerable; fatigue may prompt unexpected rest; and even weather shifts may provoke physical reactions. These are not conscious choices; they are involuntary bodily responses. At the same time, these embodied changes do not occur outside of social and cultural systems. Physical sensations and experiences are interpreted and given meaning in the context in which they are experienced. They are managed and often disciplined through a social lens that prescribes to women what they should feel, do, and avoid, reducing pregnancy to a list of standardised, depersonalised commands. Expected to exercise restraint to protect the health of their baby, compliance takes precedence over lived experience (Lupton, 2012). Between technological surveillance and rigid management protocols, women's subjective experience goes unheard, especially when caregivers work on strict time schedules.

Each of the caring professions, including medicine, nursing, and midwifery, relies on a functional understanding of the physical body that is used to indicate health or illness. In maternal healthcare, diagnostics provide critical information that can save lives and help caregivers identify and monitor potential pregnancy-related complications, enabling timely intervention when necessary. As such, they are an aspect of safe care (Hammer & Burton-Jeangros, 2013), but fall short of the mark to offer genuine understanding of a client's lived experience (Stone et al., 2022). Understanding requires practitioners who engage with clients in ways that are responsive and situated.

Beyond measurement: Reclaiming embodied knowledge

In the free-standing birth centres where this research took place, the midwife's clinical assessment of the woman, specifically her pregnant body, was part of her everyday work. Measuring the fundal height with a simple measuring tape, listening to fetal heartbeats, and palpating the baby's position were techniques used as monitoring and diagnostic tools.[1] However, these were only one aspect of a broader encounter. As I sat with Nina for her first interview in a vibrant, colourful birthing room, her enthusiasm for her new workplace spilled over. She shared stories from her first weeks of orientation, reflections that painted a picture of the chaos that comes when we are thrown into completely new circumstances. In those early weeks, with so much beginning at once, a colleague helped her turn her theoretical knowledge into a coherent practice. What had once felt like a disconnected set of tasks took shape as a new way of understanding that comprised both what she knew and what she was learning in her new work setting. One of the first appointments she observed was conducted by an experienced midwife. She told me this:

> After the appointment was over, I reflected with my colleague on how we had checked the baby. It seemed to be almost only about the mom's descriptions and sensations of her baby. Our check-up was the background to this—not the most important part because the mom was so clear. She told us quite confidently that she and her baby were both doing well; that she felt attuned to her baby; her baby was moving well; and everything was okay. Anyway, of course we did the Leopold manoeuvres [abdominal palpation]. The baby was in a head down position. The heartbeats were positive and normal, so we could check that off the list, as well. That was all good. We put together what she said about her baby with our measurements to make our assessment. And then the rest of the conversation really became about: How is she feeling at home? How is her relationship at the moment? What does it mean for her to become a mother? Is this how she imagined pregnancy would be? It's not just about prenatal care in the sense of "How is the pregnancy going?" or "Is everything developing well?"—not just the factual things you can know through measurements. It's about all of it, including her environment and how she feels in her surroundings—the mental, emotional, and physical aspects, mainly for the woman, but also for the family.
>
> *(Nina, first interview)*

This way of listening to the woman first, as was shown in Chapter 5, and placing her experience at the centre of the encounter, echoes an older tradition, one that historian Barbara Duden (1991) explored in 18th-century medical records. In her analysis, she found that 18th century physicians recorded women's descriptions of inner sensations and bodily changes, using these to arrive at a meaningful diagnosis. Listening was considered part of the diagnostic process. The women whose experiences were documented did not separate their physical symptoms from how they moved through daily life; their experience of pregnancy included descriptions of the way in which they moved through the world.

Duden (1993) draws attention to the distinction between pregnancy as something lived and pregnancy as something diagnosed and assessed. In her historical work, she highlights how the German language can demonstrate this difference more explicitly. She called these *Schwangergehen*, literally translated as *pregnant moving*, to distinguish it from *Schwangerschaft,* the word for pregnancy. *Schwangergehen* refers to moving through the world as a pregnant woman, an experience grounded in the rhythms and sensations of the body within the individual's lifeworld. It is a deeply embodied way of knowing, where the woman's own perception is foregrounded. In contrast, *Schwangerschaft*, the noun form, frames pregnancy as a physical state, one that can be confirmed and measured objectively.

By the end of the Enlightenment, medical knowledge had shifted away from lived experience of the patient and moved towards standardisation and quantification. Early German obstetric texts reveal physicians' unease with women's self-described signs of pregnancy (Schlumbohm, 2002), since individual accounts of pregnancy were often regarded as unreliable and thought to lack diagnostic value (Borkowsky, 1988; Fasbender, 1906/1964). Medical reasoning, shaped by inductive logic, came to privilege what the physician could observe and verify through his own senses, thereby diminishing the relevance of the patient's own account (Hampson, 1968/1990).

As obstetrics became institutionalised, women's subjective experiences completely lost authority (Davis-Floyd, 1994), evident in how pregnancy is diagnosed. Instead of relying on women's physical changes, a second line on a test strip, a hormone value in a blood sample, or a digital image on a screen takes precedence. These diagnostics are seen as providing fact-based, impartial information, and it is taken for granted that they constitute the only basis for diagnosis. A woman's own sensations are no longer required because they are not hard facts (Rothman, 1986/1993). The use of ultrasound technology to look inside the womb has also replaced women's accounts of fetal movement, altering how they connect to their developing baby (Stone et al., 2022). Whereas a woman's report of her baby's first movements, also called quickening, was once a sure sign of pregnancy, these movements are now first seen on a screen, often weeks before they are physically felt (Lupton, 2013; Mitchell, 2001). In this clinical model, embodied knowledge is undervalued and routinely displaced by technologies that privilege the visual and the measurable.

Learning abdominal palpation

Abdominal palpation, often referred to as the Leopold manoeuvres, is a hands-on method used by midwives and clinicians to assess the position, presentation, and engagement of the fetal presenting part during pregnancy. It involves a sequence of systematic palpation (touches) of the pregnant woman's abdomen to identify fetal parts. As described in the literature (Nishikawa & Sakakibara, 2013; Stone et al., 2022; Walker & Sabrosa, 2014), this practice is both diagnostic and relational; it provides clinical information while also inviting connection between the midwife, woman, and baby. For the newly qualified midwives, palpation was a technique that enabled them to come into contact with the lived body of their clients, a practice largely absent from their clinical training. During their orientation in their free-standing birth centre, they began to 'see' and 'listen' inside the womb with their hands, sensing form, movement, and tension. Tactile listening supported embodied perception. As they gained experience providing antenatal care in their free-standing birth centre, they began to trust their hands and were, over time, able to integrate this with their theoretical knowledge. In doing so, they entered into a dialogue with the woman's embodied presence, allowing them to dwell more fully in the encounter.

Most of the newly qualified midwives had not had extensive practical experience with abdominal palpation during their clinical training and needed time at the beginning of their orientation to improve their skills. During my first interview with Nanette, she shifted in her chair and glanced away before she began to speak, hesitant to share what still felt like an uncomfortable memory from her early weeks during her orientation.

What's my experience of the Leopolds? Well, it's gotten better, but at the beginning I always had this feeling—oh God. First I'd think, okay, that could be the back [of the baby]. Then I'd keep palpating and think—no, that can't be it. Always this back and forth, always this switching. It could be here, it could be there. And then I wouldn't know anymore—no idea at all. And then yes, I'd listen to the fetal heartbeats, and that would help a little, not always, but then I'd think—okay, maybe I did get it right, but I still couldn't say with 100% certainty that what I felt was the back. Then, one of my colleagues said to me: Why don't you go with your first thought about what it is? And that was the turning point where I thought—actually, yes. Just go with the first answer you have—trust it. Then, I'd listen again—hear the fetal heartbeats in the spot where I had palpated the back of the baby, and, most of the time, it was accurate. Of course, I still make mistakes. I think the back is on the left and it turns out it was on the right. I always ask a colleague for confirmation if I'm uncertain. So, I've become more confident. But it's this process of translating something spatial—something that can't be seen—into what you feel with your hands. You have to trust in your hands and let the image take form.

(Nanette, first interview)

Learning to translate touch into a spatial picture was deeply moving for the newly qualified midwives, even as it became routine, making the body more than just a neutral site to be processed and assessed. Women bring with them their personal history, an identity, a set of cultural expectations, and often, the pros and cons of medicalised surveillance. As human beings, we all have a layered presence. When carrying out abdominal palpation, these distinct but overlapping layers were revealed. According to Scheper-Hughes and Lock (1987), the individual body (as lived experience), the social body (as a symbol for society and its norms), and the body politic (as regulated by institutions and systems of power) represent distinct and interconnected ways of understanding the body. For midwives, learning to recognise and respond to this complexity meant moving beyond the clinical gaze and embracing touch as a way of seeing and listening differently.

As newly qualified midwives became more confident in performing the Leopold manoeuvres, something else began to shift. Abdominal palpation became a way of slowing down and entering into shared presence. Toni shared her experience with me:

I think palpating the pregnant woman's belly is the most beautiful moment [in antenatal care] because I'm really in contact with the woman and her baby and I can feel how a relationship between us is getting built—differently than if we are only talking with each other. For example, if I only ask a woman: how are you? — then the conversation remains rather superficial. But, if I ask her something more personal, such as asking her to tell me about her first birth, then a closeness develops between us just through her telling and my listening. The women get more emotional when they talk about a personal event rather than just staying on the surface with the question: How are you? When a woman talks about her first birth, she begins to feel her memories, and I can connect with her through her feelings. After that, I ask her to lie down and ask: "May I touch your belly?" And then when that touch happens—I have the feeling that, if you're speaking at the same time—talking about the baby, about the movement—it becomes like a bridge. There's a connection with the woman— different somehow. I remember the woman better when I've touched her than if I just sat across from her at the table during an appointment. Then I also know: I touched that woman. We have a connection. We've shared something. It's a deeper experience.

(Toni, first interview)

Through abdominal palpation, midwifery, particularly in free-standing birth centres, offers a counterpoint to clinical care, which predominantly privileges what can be measured. During palpation, midwives speak with the woman and the baby. Whispering "hello" before beginning the Leopold manoeuvres, while a seemingly small gesture, changes the meaning of the encounter. Amelia expressed her process for engaging the pregnant woman and the baby, clearly inviting the baby to take part in the interaction.

> I talk to the baby when I do the Leopold manoeuvres. I usually only touch the pregnant woman once they say they're ready. I don't ask: "May I touch you?" but rather: "Let me know when you're ready for me to touch you." That's what I do. And then to the baby, I usually say: "Hello, baby." And then something like: "It's me, Amelia, we already know each other." Or: "We don't know each other yet." And then—well—toward the end of the pregnancy, when it's getting closer to the birth, I'll say something like: "Hey, we're really excited. You can start making your way to us if you're ready."— if it's around the due date, something like that. And earlier in the pregnancy, I don't talk to the baby for a long time. I just introduce myself and sometimes say what I'm about to do—that I want to measure and palpate and listen to the heartbeat—um—and maybe ask if it feels like moving around a little and greeting both me and mom.
>
> *(Amelia, first interview)*

Rather than reducing care to a series of measurable outputs, Amelia's interaction invited the possibility of what Hermann Schmitz calls a *resonance field*: a dynamic space of mutual sensing in which bodies adjust, respond, and reveal themselves to one another, eliciting knowledge through relationship (2019). Touch becomes a medium for relational depth; a quiet form of listening in which the body speaks and is heard. Skeide, in her praxiography of home birth, wrote:

> The midwife's and the woman's bodies, but also the midwife's and the child's bodies, get increasingly familiar with each other through touching and feeling, and becoming familiar authorizes a more detailed obstetrical examination of the child. When diagnosing is combined with getting to know each other, relating personally and intimately helps to do better diagnostics.
>
> *(2019, p. 244)*

This mode of practice demands what Benner (1984) terms embodied expertise, a form of knowing that arises from immersion, experience, and responsiveness.

At a time when maternity care is increasingly mediated by technologies that distance clinicians from the embodied realities of those they care for, these descriptions offer an important reminder: clinical information, however accurate, does not in itself yield understanding. Technologies may register signals, but they cannot initiate or replace a relationship. The midwife's hands can help cultivate meaning and trust, so that shared knowledge can emerge. Metaphorically, Echo is nourished, able to regain her voice and interact meaningfully. In this way, midwifery reclaims not only the practice of touch, but its ontological significance.

Questions for reflection

1 When you practice abdominal palpation, how do you experience the interaction? Do you wait for the baby to respond to you?
2 How do you navigate moments of uncertainty in clinical care? What strategies help you stay grounded when you are uncertain, for example, during abdominal palpation?
3 Can you recall a time when wonder shaped your understanding of the body or your relationship with a client? How did you share or process that experience?
4 What does the term *lived body* mean in your personal or professional life? How does it differ from the clinical body?
5 How do you listen—not just with your ears, but with your hands, your attention, or your whole body?

Note

1 In Germany, midwives in free-standing birth centres very rarely conduct ultrasound diagnostic.

References

Benner, P. (1984). *From Novice to Expert, Excellence and Power in Clinical Nursing Practice*. Prentice Hall.

Berg, M., & Harterink, P. (2004). Embodying the patient: Records and bodies in early 20th-century US medical practice. *Body Soc, 10*(2–3), 13–41.

Borkowsky, M. (1988). *Krankheit Schwangerschaft?: Schwangerschaft, Geburt und Wochenbett aus ärztlicher Sicht seit 1800* [Disease Pregnancy? Pregnancy, Birth and the Post Partum Period from the perspective of doctors since 1800]. Chronos.

Davis-Floyd, R. (1994). The technocratic body: American childbirth as cultural expression. *Soc Sci Med, 38*(8), 1125–1140.

Descartes, R. (2007). *Discourse on Method* (P. Kraus & F. Hunt, Eds.). Focus Publishing.

Drew, N. (1986). Exclusion and confirmation: A phenomenology of patients' experiences with caregivers. *J Nurs Scholarsh, 18*(2), 39–43. https://doi.org/10.1111/j.1547-5069.1986.tb00540.x

Duden, B. (1991). *The Woman Beneath the Skin: A Doctor's Patients in Eighteenth-Century Germany*. Harvard University Press.

Duden, B. (1993). *Disembodying Women: Perspectives on Pregnancy and the Unborn*. Harvard University Press.

Fasbender, H. (1906/1964). *Geschichte der Geburtshilfe* [History of Obstetrics] (Nachdr. d. Ausg. Jena 1906 ed.). Olms.

Goldstein, K. (1934). *Der aufbau des organismus; einführung in die biologie unter besonderer berücksichtigung der erfahrungen am kranken menschen*. M. Mijhof.

Hammer, R. P., & Burton-Jeangros, C. (2013, Sep). Tensions around risks in pregnancy: A typology of women's experiences of surveillance medicine. *Soc Sci Med, 93*, 55–63. https://doi.org/10.1016/j.socscimed.2013.05.033

Hampson, N. (1968/1990). *The Enlightenment*. Penguin Books.

Lupton, D. (1994/2012). *Medicine as Culture: Illness, Disease and the Body* (3rd ed.) [Kindle]. Sage. https://doi.org/10.4135/9781446254530

Lupton, D. (2012). 'Precious cargo': Foetal subjects, risk and reproductive citizenship. *Crit Public Health, 22*(3), 329–340. https://doi.org/10.1080/09581596.2012.657612

Lupton, D. (2013). Quantifying the body: Monitoring and measuring health in the age of mHealth technologies. *Crit Public Health, 23*(4), 393–403. https://doi.org/10.1080/09581596.2013.794931

Merleau-Ponty, M. (1958). *Phenomenology of Perception* (C. Smith, Trans.). Routledge Classics.

Mitchell, L. M. (2001). *Baby's First Picture: Ultrasound and the Politics of Fetal Subjects.* University of Toronto Press.

Nishikawa, M., & Sakakibara, H. (2013, Feb 19). Effect of nursing intervention program using abdominal palpation of Leopold's maneuvers on maternal-fetal attachment. *Reprod Health, 10*, 12. https://doi.org/10.1186/1742-4755-10-12

Ovid. (2004). *Metamorphoses* (C. Martin, Trans.; Electronic ed.). W.W. Norton & Company.

Rothman, B. K. (1986/1993). *The Tentative Pregnancy: Prenatal Diagnosis and the Future of Motherhood.* Norton Paperback.

Scheper-Hughes, N., & Lock, M. M. (1987). The mindful body: A prolegomenon to medical anthropology. *Med Anthropol Q, 1*(1), 6–41. https://www.jstor.org/stable/648769

Schlumbohm, J. (2002). *Verhandlungen zwischen Arzt und Schwangeren im Entbindungsshospital der Universität Göttingen um 1800* [Negotiations between doctor and pregnant women at a maternity hospital at the university of Göttigen around 1800]. Vandenhoeck & Ruprecht.

Schmitz, H. (2019). *New Phenomenology: A Brief Introduction.* Mimesis International.

Skeide, A. (2019, Jun). Enacting homebirth bodies: Midwifery techniques in Germany. *Cult Med Psychiatry, 43*(2), 236–255. https://doi.org/10.1007/s11013-018-9613-8

Stone, N. I., Downe, S., Dykes, F., & Rothman, B. K. (2022, Jan). "Putting the baby back in the body": The re-embodiment of pregnancy to enhance safety in a free-standing birth center. *Midwifery, 104*, 103172. https://doi.org/10.1016/j.midw.2021.103172

Walker, S., & Sabrosa, R. (2014). Assessment of fetal presentation: Exploring a woman-centred approach. *Br J Midwifery, 22*(4). https://doi.org/10.12968/bjom.2014.22.4.240

7

"I'VE ARRIVED." WELCOMING BABIES INTO THE WORLD

Introduction

In Chapter 6, we explored how newly qualified midwives developed their embodied expertise through the use of abdominal palpation. In this chapter, we reflect on the notion of *arrival* and what this means in terms of birth. In addition to this, across newly qualified midwives' stories, there was a shared understanding that arrival also carried the meaning of being recognised as a midwife and feeling a part of the team.

Arrival: Welcoming babies into the world

The word "arrival" has its roots in the language of sea travel. The Latin *arripare*, meaning "to touch the shore," evokes the concrete image of a ship reaching land after time at sea. In contemporary English, arrival can refer to a person reaching a destination or achieving recognition, or even to the launch of a product. For example, in the age of technology, the arrival of products such as smartphones on the market is celebrated with spectacular events. However, in ordinary life, arrival is rarely that conspicuous. Humans are arriving all the time, into rooms, conversations, relationships, and tasks, usually without taking conscious notice of the subtle changes that occur in body language, awareness, and mood.

The concept of arrival also has metaphorical underpinnings. Beyond its meaning of reaching a physical destination, it can also evoke an inner sense of settling in. It gestures towards a process of being well received within a given world. In its most existential sense, the first arrival for every human being is their birth—their arrival in the world. This moment is biologically primal, while at the same time shaped by culture and emotion. The newborn, considered at its most vulnerable

DOI: 10.4324/9781003591306-7

and utterly dependent for its transition on the conditions into which it is received, is welcomed by a constellation of others: midwives, physicians, partners, and kin. I refer to these as the *arrival committee*, a term that includes structure, protocol, and presence.

In the clinical sense, for a newborn to have arrived well means that it has successfully adapted to extrauterine life within the first minutes after birth. This physiological transition primarily involves changes in the respiratory and cardiovascular systems. With the first breath, the alveoli in the lungs expand, allowing the infant to take in air and begin gas exchange in an oxygen-rich environment. Simultaneously, the fetal circulatory shunts, such as the ductus arteriosus, the ductus venosus, and the foramen ovale, begin to close, redirecting blood flow through the lungs so that oxygenation can occur independently of the placenta. This physical adaptation is paramount.

In many cultures, the birth of a baby is also a deeply symbolic moment that marks the infant's entry into a specific social and cultural world. The ways in which newborns are welcomed vary widely and often reflect core values and cosmologies. In Ethiopia, among the Macha Galla, it is customary for women to leave their husband's village and return to their parents' home for the birth of their first two children (Bartels, 1969). As they are still considered newcomers in their husband's village, a degree of mistrust remains, leaving both mother and infant exposed to possible spiritual harm. To protect against this, the women travel back to their natal home in the company of two, four, or six female companions from their husband's village. These companions bring food and gifts but do not stay for the birth itself. As the birth nears, fragrant wood is burned, and fresh grass is laid on the floor in a specially prepared room where the woman will give birth. Once the baby is born, the attending women ululate to announce the birth, signalling the baby's sex by the number of cries: four for a girl, five for a boy. These ritual gestures form part of a wider cultural practice that marks birth as both a physical and spiritual transition, a structured arrival into family and village life.

Among Hindu birth customs, which vary according to the caste a baby is born into, the Jatakarma ceremony is a significant rite that is often performed at birth to welcome the newborn into the family (Gatrad et al., 2004). During this ritual, the father touches and smells the child, whispering sacred mantras into the infant's ears. These gestures are meant to ensure a safe and spiritually grounded entrance into the world. Additionally, protective symbols like a black dot or the sacred Om may be drawn behind the baby's ear or placed on a necklace to ward off evil. These customs venerate birth as both a physical and metaphysical transition, underscored by ritual care.

In Nunavik, northern Quebec, Inuit communities have reclaimed birth as a central part of cultural identity and community healing (Van Wagner et al., 2007). After decades of evacuating pregnant women to southern hospitals, a practice experienced as disempowering and culturally disruptive, Inuit midwives re-established local birthing practices through the Inuulitsivik midwifery model. Community-based birth centres provide a space for blending traditional knowledge with clinical practice, supported by training methods imbued with cultural practices such as storytelling and reflection. The birthplace allows babies to be born amongst kin, each baby celebrated by adding their footprint to a wall that links maternity care to community life. In these contexts, birth is not just a clinical event, but an act of cultural continuity and autonomy. As reflected in these descriptions, some customs are place-dependent, while others can be carried out discreetly in a hospital labour ward.

Learning to restructure the arrival of the baby: Birth in free-standing birth centres

In contrast to the welcoming traditions in numerous cultures throughout the world, student midwives are taught a range of clinical procedures to be carried out at the time of birth. These may include assisting the woman into the lithotomy position, positioning the birth companion at the head of the bed, calling for a second midwife or obstetrician, and performing immediate newborn care measures. Such measures often include placing the baby on the mother's chest, suctioning the newborn's airways, drying the infant, and clamping the umbilical cord, either immediately after birth or waiting until pulsation has ceased, called delayed cord clamping. These interventions are shaped by institutional norms, clinical guidelines, and the local culture of care within birth settings. Even though the social and symbolic dimensions of a baby's arrival carry deep meaning for the family, in midwifery education, the role of the arrival committee as the carriers of culture in the welcoming of a newborn is rarely extended beyond the clinical procedures.

The newly qualified midwives often left me voice messages following births that stirred strong emotions. One newly qualified midwife, Annabelle, shared an experience in which she described the first birth she observed at her birth centre. Her early orientation period differed from the other newly qualified midwives, who began observing births within the first six weeks of their orientation. In contrast, Annabelle focused exclusively on antenatal appointments and postpartum home visits for the first six months. By the time she began attending births, she had already met all the women registered to give birth at the centre and felt a strong sense of familiarity with them.

Annabelle took particular interest in reflecting on how the theoretical concepts she had studied translated into practice. She approached this process methodically, often comparing her practical experiences with the theories and constructs she had encountered during her education. Although she had learned about the concept of bonding and its significance for both mother and baby, she had never fully grasped what it meant in practice. She left me the following message after observing her first birth in her free-standing birth centre:

I was at an amazing birth two days ago and witnessed something totally new for me. After the woman gave birth, the midwife passed the baby to the mom, who couldn't take her eyes off him. I could see her falling in love! For the first time, I saw what bonding actually looks like. I was mesmerised. She dried him off with a towel and spoke to him in a quiet, loving voice. It really moved me.

(Annabelle, voice message 2)[1]

Birth, in a metaphorical sense, marks the separation of the woman from her baby after having been joined for the duration of the pregnancy. The period directly after birth begins a new process in which mother and baby encounter one another as separate beings, gradually forming a new, earthly connection through touch, gaze, scent, and sound. This early phase of bonding is not only physical and emotional, but also relational and culturally mediated, shaped by the ways in which a society, institution, or religion structures and interprets the first moments of life. For Annabelle, this moment of bonding revealed something she had only known as a theoretical construct during her studies. She had never seen a woman gaze at her newborn with such tenderness in an act of reunification after birth. In her clinical education, she was taught to place the baby immediately on the mother's chest, before the mother had a chance to really look at her child and take in the miracle that had just occurred. At this birth, she witnessed what she now recognised as woman-led or embodied bonding, something that had existed for her only as an abstract idea until that moment.

Annabelle told me the story of this birth again during her second interview. In the retelling of this birth story, her focus was on how the midwife made this baby's arrival so special.

I told you about this birth in a voice message. It was my first birth at the birth centre. I basically just sat in the corner and observed. I listened closely to everything my colleague said to the couple—her exact words. It's so much different than what I heard in my clinical training. Another thing that was really different is that this woman was getting up and moving around intuitively without asking anyone for permission. I was trying to digest what this meant on a deeper level, especially after the baby was born. This was so different than what I had witnessed and learned as a student. At this birth, after the baby was born, the midwife was really patient—it was as if she was able to slow down time and let everything unfold at its own pace. She was so relaxed. I found it amazing that my colleague could take 15 minutes to do what I was supposed to do in under 5 minutes in the clinic. The most mind-blowing part was that the actual tasks were the same ones that we did in the hospital—but the slow pace changed everything.

(Annabelle, second interview)[2]

Moments like this were intentionally curated by the experienced midwives with a mood of reverence and respect, to give the mother time to discover her baby visually and tactilely. As is evident in this story, this did not just support the baby's arrival; it also marked a kind of arrival for Annabelle in terms of her future professional responsibilities.

Arrival, disclosure, and appropriation

In Heideggerian terms, when something previously concealed is revealed through an event or experience, it is often accompanied by a shift in understanding (Stone & Thomson, 2025). For Annabelle, witnessing that first birth changed her perspective of labouring women, as well as her understanding of the midwife's role directly after birth. She did not merely observe a birth; she arrived in her own practice, entering into a midwifery philosophy that values time, presence, and awe. Performing the necessary tasks to support a newborn's adaptation to extrauterine life is just one aspect of midwifery care. Equally important is an attentiveness to temporality, a sensitivity to the pace at which the relationship between mother and child begins to grow in the moments after birth, as space is held for reunion and bonding.

These kinds of experiential shifts marked key moments in the professional becoming of the newly qualified midwives. However, while experiences of awe and joy were most intense at births, their sense of having arrived did not always unfold in exciting moments, but often in mundane, daily interactions. As the newly qualified midwives began to settle into the everyday rhythm in their birth centre, a different kind of arrival took shape, one that shifted their understanding and deepened both their sense of professional identity and belonging.

Arriving at the workplace

While births offered newly qualified midwives moments of awe and existential recognition, a different form of arrival took place within the routines of daily practice, in which moments of identification and acknowledgement sparked a shift in identity. These seemingly ordinary acts carried symbolic weight, affirming the midwife's arrival through both the tasks she performed and her growing sense of belonging within the team, signalling to her that she was becoming a midwife in her own right. This deeper sense of arrival came at different moments for each newly qualified midwife. Sheila described how meaningful it was for her to finally have appointments of her own with pregnant clients:

> At the beginning, I had to follow the other midwives. I just went along with them. The whole situation was so new and surreal. That meant that every evening I would check: Okay, what appointments are scheduled for tomorrow? Where can I tag along? And that really stressed me out—not being able to schedule anything myself. And I think the main issue was that I felt like I was just joining in on the appointments and not running them myself, not leading the conversations with the women. The moment that changed, I felt: Okay, yes. I've arrived as a midwife in the birth centre, and I'm not just a student midwife tagging along.
>
> *(Sheila, first interview)*

In this moment, Sheila no longer saw herself as someone temporarily present or dependent on other midwives. Conducting antenatal appointments independently and being seen as the responsible midwife marked a shift in how she understood herself, as well as how others related to her.

Toni described a moment of acknowledgement when the midwife on call asked her to come to a birth at the birth centre. Her voice message, sent just after a birth, expressed a sense of belonging, joy, and gratitude:

> So, I'll just tell you now because I've just come from my first birth at the birth centre, and everything is still settling. Earlier I was just glowing, elated—and I still am. I'm walking through the streets with a smile on my face, on my way home, and I'm really, really happy that I'm finally feeling a sense of having arrived at the birth centre. Now I'm part of everything that takes place there. I am so grateful that the colleagues think of me when it comes to births, that they call me in—that's such a good feeling. And I really got to observe a dream birth to start with. A first-time mom who gave birth just like in the textbook—but not the hospital textbook. It was beautiful and very calm. The midwife didn't need to do a vaginal exam, because it was completely clear just from how the woman was moving and what she was doing that things were progressing. For a first birth, it went pretty quickly. I was at the birth centre at 3 a.m. and the baby was born shortly after 7. It was just lovely. I can feel I'm still in the phase of figuring out where I fit in. I was there as the third midwife, and that gave me a certain sense of security. I'm still totally glowing and just happy—and it was so sweet how the couple explicitly thanked me at the end. That really does something to you. That was really a moment of: Yes, I was there, I was part of it. I made the right decision to work here.
>
> *(Toni, voice message 1)*

Being seen and acknowledged by both colleagues and clients was central to Toni's experience of arrival. Even with limited responsibility as the third midwife, she felt appreciated, as if her presence had carried meaning for others. These small gestures of recognition, while seemingly minor, were nevertheless formative. The next excerpt shows how external confirmation could come through something as simple as writing one's name in the client's record booklet.

> I had the feeling I had arrived when I wrote my name in a client's record booklet for the first time, under the birth centre's stamp. That was so beautiful. I still remember exactly when I did this for the first time. A colleague was sitting next to me. I was about to hand the booklet back to the woman when the colleague said: Wait, you have to write your name and phone number there. That was the first time my name appeared as the primary midwife in official documents, so that anyone who looks inside it knows: okay, she's being looked after by me—I'm her midwife. That was incredible.
>
> *(Nina, first interview)*

Here, the gesture of writing a name is not only administrative. It affirms account-ability and relational commitment, signalling a shift from student to responsible midwife. The final story about arrival was told by Sally at a later stage in her orientation:

> This week I had a birth during the night leading into Friday, and I went straight to the partnership meeting afterward to sign my contract with the team. They had given their approval! I had worked all night and hadn't slept at all. We had a check-in round and I said, I feel like I've been welcomed into such a lovely midwifery team, and I've finally arrived. I was so moved that I cried. It was such a beautiful moment.
>
> *(Sally, second interview)*

While signing a contract is a common, formal milestone, in this case she experi-enced it as collective recognition from her team.

Such moments seem modest in outward appearance, yet they revealed the phe-nomenon of arrival in a deeper, ontological sense. They constituted what Heidegger refers to as *Ereignis*, an event in which being is appropriated by [the]world, and something previously concealed is disclosed as meaningful (Polt, 2005; Stone & Thomson, 2025). In these instances, the newly qualified midwives suddenly found themselves positioned differently. They were no longer an observer or assistant, for they had arrived at a fuller sense of their presence as a midwife.

Heidegger's (1962/2001) notion of *Lichtung*, or clearing, also offers a compel-ling lens through which to view these experiences. *Clearing* refers to the opening in which beings can appear as they are, a space of disclosure where understanding becomes possible (Smythe & Spence, 2020). Arrival, in this context, denotes a shift in understanding, where one's role is not only enacted but inhabited. What was pre-viously abstract, whether clinical knowledge, professional identity, or the relational ethos of midwifery, becomes one's own. These events, while grounded in the con-crete practices of midwifery, were moments of ontological transformation. They were experiences in which the midwives' identity and practice were reconfigured.

In this sense, *arrival* does not merely follow *seeing the whole* in a linear sequence. It deepens and completes it. The newly qualified midwife, no longer standing outside the scene she is trying to comprehend, becomes part of its unfold-ing. What began as observation, quite literally standing outside the bubble, becomes embodied belonging. Arrival marks the moment when seeing the whole begins to feel "lived," and practice starts to take root in the midwife's evolving sense of her developing professional identity.

Questions for reflection

1 How do you understand the meaning of *arrival*, both in terms of a baby being born and your own emergence as a midwife or caregiver? What moments shaped this understanding for you?

2 In what ways have you experienced or witnessed bonding as something more than a clinical recommendation? How does this shape your approach to the early moments after birth?

3 Describe the look in the parents' eyes when they see their baby for the first time.

4 What practices or gestures have you seen or taken part in that made a baby's arrival special rather than simply managed? What made these moments stand out?

5 How have seemingly ordinary acts (like being called in to assist or writing your name in documentation) influenced your sense of professional identity and belonging?

Notes

1 A different version of this quote from Annabelle was previously published in: Stone, N. I., & Thomson, G. (2025). Exploring newly qualified midwives' lived experiences of out-of-hospital births through voice messaging and interviews. *Int J Qual Methods*, 24, 1–16. https://doi.org/10.1177/16094069251346849.

2 A different version of this quote from Annabelle was previously published in Stone, N. I., & Thomson, G. (2025). Exploring newly qualified midwives' lived experiences of out-of-hospital births through voice messaging and interviews. *Int J Qual Methods*, 24, 1–16. https://doi.org/10.1177/16094069251346849.

References

Bartels, L. (1969). Birth customs and birth songs of the Macha Galla. *Ethnol, 8*(4), 406–422. https://www.jstor.org/stable/3772909

Gatrad, A. R., Ray, M., & Sheikh, A. (2004, Dec). Hindu birth customs. *Arch Dis Child, 89*(12), 1094–1097. https://doi.org/10.1136/adc.2004.050591

Heidegger, M. (1962/2001). *Being and Time* (J. Macquarrie & E. S. Robinson, Trans.; 7th ed.). Blackwell Publishers.

Polt, R. (2005). Ereignis. In H. L. Dreyfus & M. A. Wrathall (Eds.), *A Companion to Heidegger (Blackwell Companions to Philosophy)* (Kindle ed.). *23*, 6741–7046. Blackwell Publishing Ltd.

Smythe, E., & Spence, D. (2020, Apr). Reading Heidegger. *Nurs Philos, 21*(2), e12271. https://doi.org/10.1111/nup.12271

Stone, N. I., & Thomson, G. (2025). Exploring newly qualified midwives' lived experiences of out-of-hospital births through voice messaging and interviews. *Int J Qual Methods, 24*, 1–16. https://doi.org/10.1177/16094069251346849

Van Wagner, V., Epoo, B., Nastapoka, J., & Harney, E. (2007, Jul-Aug). Reclaiming birth, health, and community: Midwifery in the inuit villages of Nunavik, Canada. *J Midwifery Womens Health, 52*(4), 384–391. https://doi.org/10.1016/j.jmwh.2007.03.025

8

"THEY'RE MOTIVATED AND WILLING TO WORK HARD." EXPERIENCED MIDWIVES' LIVED EXPERIENCE OF NEWLY QUALIFIED MIDWIVES' ORIENTATION

Introduction

In Chapter 7, we explored how newly qualified midwives experienced a sense of arrival as midwives and as recognised members of their birth centre team. These moments of arrival often emerged through small yet significant shifts in identity, when they gained acknowledgement from both colleagues and clients or when they encountered in practice what had previously existed for them only as an abstract theoretical construct. In this chapter, we turn to the focus group interviews, in which the experienced midwives shared their lived experience of supporting newly qualified midwives during their orientation. This chapter highlights how relational competence, communication, and integration in the team were equally vital to newly qualified midwives' orientation as their clinical skill and knowledge acquisition.

Integration, socialisation, and disciplinary technologies

To understand the process of transitioning from hospital care to care in free-standing birth centres and home births, it is essential to consider how socialisation and integration shape the learning process. Becoming a midwife involves more than just acquiring theoretical and practical knowledge; it also requires adapting to the shared culture and professional norms of midwifery as it is practiced in the new setting. Benoit et al. (2001, p. 139) distinguish between midwifery education, referring to the formal requirements of training, and socialisation, which is the informal process through which midwives absorb the values, procedures, and traditions of the profession. Ivan Illich, philosopher, critic, and historian, called this *hidden curriculum* (1973 in Benoit et al., 2001, p. 139), emphasising how unspoken norms and expectations shape professional identity. Before standardised midwifery

DOI: 10.4324/9781003591306-8

education, midwives learned their skills and knowledge through apprenticeship training. Rather than studying theoretical concepts and adjusting to institutional protocols, they learned by observing and working alongside an experienced midwife. Through apprenticeship, they absorbed the customs of the villages where they trained, becoming intimately familiar with local families, their kinship structures, and histories (Labouvie, 2007). Because they trained in the same settings where they would eventually practice, they were already socialised into the community and integrated into their role as a midwife.

Surtees (2008), in her research on transitioning from student to midwife, examined how so-called disciplinary technologies shaped the experiences of newly qualified midwives in Aotearoa/New Zealand. Disciplinary technologies, as described by philosopher Michel Foucault (1977), are ways in which institutions like schools, hospitals, and workplaces guide and shape individual behaviour through routines, norms, and expectations. Rather than relying on direct control, these techniques encourage people to regulate themselves in accordance with the standards of the community they are learning and working in. Drawing on Foucauldian discourse analysis, Surtees explored how midwifery education outwardly focusses on developing clinical skills, while masking a hidden agenda that promotes the internalisation of institutional norms. In her study, individuals who, through training and surveillance, learned to conform to institutional expectations, did not require direct coercion to behave and work as expected. In midwifery education, this occurs through constant assessment, structured feedback, and hierarchical oversight, where students absorb the spoken and unspoken rules of the hospital system and unconsciously modify their behaviours to align with the dominant authority (Surtees, 2008).

Tara, a newly qualified midwife, had an experience which reflects Surtees' findings. Tara shared her experience with me:

What is taught in school is kind of like this: Well, I think it doesn't actually come from the academic classes we had but happens during our clinical placements. For example, a woman comes into the hospital, gets hooked up to the fetal heart monitor, and we have to make sure that both the woman and the baby are doing well. In the back of our minds, it's always like: Something could be wrong. And I think, ugh, I really have to control myself, to stay positive and to recognize the right moment: when is there actually an emergency? Maybe that's something that just can't be taught in school. No idea. And it shouldn't be like that because I'm actually so proud to be working in the birth centre now and not in some dreadful hospital where I have to go to an early shift, worried about whether I'm doing everything right. That fear that I felt at the birth centre in the first two weeks—I realize now—was definitely there from clinical training. I was so afraid that someone was looking over my shoulder and would reprimand me at any moment. Instead, I can just be—you know—just be me.

You know, the way things were during training—why was that so accepted? It's such a horrible hospital hierarchy. It's disgusting. As a student, you have to jump in and go along with it. Even though you actually don't want to, even though you have different ideas, or you're naive, and then you arrive and just get stomped into the ground. And yeah, okay, then you have to fight your way back up and work your way through it. At the large university hospital where I did part of my training, it was even harder.

(Tara, first interview)

As Tara explained, midwifery students learn to monitor and regulate their clinical practice, often adapting their approach to fit within hospital standards and hierarchies, even when these conflict with the philosophy of woman-centred care that originally attracted them to the profession.

Ruth Surtees' (2008) study underscores how the midwifery system of education that she researched was structured around institutional oversight and medical authority, requiring newly qualified midwives to continuously negotiate their professional autonomy when they transitioned after their education. These dynamics were also visible in my data. While the free-standing birth centres fostered a more relational and less hierarchical environment than is common in most hospital settings, certain norms and expectations still guided how newly qualified midwives were evaluated and socialised into the team. The following account, shared by an experienced midwife, illustrates how observational practices and subtle forms of behavioural alignment functioned within the birth centre context:

Zoe: I know that being observed creates a certain kind of tension for our new colleagues, but it's the only way we can truly get a sense of how they work. When I'm with a new team member, I pay attention to her documentation and how she performs the Leopold manoeuvres [abdominal palpation]. Now that I know our newest colleague better, I'd say that—even though she was visibly tense during antenatal appointments—she still stayed connected and spoke with a calm, clear voice. That was remarkable in and of itself. But what really stood out to me was hearing her use expressions that she had clearly picked up from one of our more experienced colleagues. For example, our colleague Anna has been with us for a long time, and she always says to clients before she does abdominal palpation: "I'm going to touch your hand first, so you know the temperature of my hand, and then I'll touch your belly." At the appointment where I was observing our new[ly qualified] midwife, I heard her say exactly the same thing, and I remember having thought—ah, that's Anna's influence. It felt like Anna was in the room with us.

(Team 6, focus group interview)

The act of borrowing language from a respected colleague served as a sign of learning, as well as functioning as a way to demonstrate belonging. From a Foucauldian point of view, one might argue that disciplinary technologies were at work here as well, albeit in a more compassionate form.

While Foucault's framework highlights institutional discipline, Lave and Wenger (1991) offer a more practice-oriented lens, viewing integration not as regulation but as participation within a community of practice. Learning is seen as part of a social activity whereby newcomers take on characteristics of their mentors. Lave and Wenger (1991, p. 29) have written that *[L]earners inevitably participate in communities of practitioners and ... the mastery of knowledge and skill requires newcomers to move toward full participation in the socio-cultural practices of a community.* Lave and Wenger (1991) developed the term legitimate peripheral participation to explain how skills are learned, as well as to describe how a community recreates itself by passing on knowledge in its own particular way.

Verbal and non-verbal communication at births

Each free-standing birth centre I visited had its own distinctive character. While clinical guidelines were consistent throughout the free-standing birth centres I visited, the organisation of the teams and the way they coordinated care varied. Newly qualified midwives in this study therefore encountered similar situational learning experiences and achieved a similar scope of skill and knowledge acquisition, but the rhythm and structure of orientation differed depending on the team dynamic. This included team size, the number of annual births, and whether care was shared across the team or divided into smaller caseload teams within the larger team.

While the orientation process was meant to support skill and knowledge acquisition, what came into view consistently across sites was the significance of learning to communicate and understand emotional and relational cues to establish trusting relationships with clients and colleagues. In several focus groups, midwives described how uncomfortable it is to work with a new colleague with whom they cannot yet communicate effectively, whether verbally or non-verbally. Perfect communication is not expected from the beginning; it does, however, serve as an indicator as to whether a new colleague is ready to take on additional responsibilities without oversight. In one focus group, the experienced midwives reflected together on their experiences of communicating with newly qualified midwives:

Sophia: It makes a difference if you work at a birth with a familiar colleague or with someone new to the team. With a new colleague, you just have to lock eyes with her, and you know she's still new to her role here and not completely present. You don't need to hash that out in detail—you can read it in her eyes.

Elena: The old hands don't need words to know what the other is thinking. We just look at each other. Especially you two—and maybe Yolanda as well—we've always worked that way. We always know what the other is thinking. It's written all over their face.

Sophia: And that's a different kind of working together than with brand-new midwives. Absolutely.

Linda: I don't trust a new colleague to work alone until she can read a situation and communicate it. I need to know that she understands what's happening.

Elena: I think it starts with verbal communication. I'm thinking of two completely different births, both with newly qualified midwives. Both were in the large birthing room, and both involved postpartum haemorrhages. I was the backup for the new midwife, so there were three midwives at the birth. With the first birth, I noticed that she suddenly froze right after the baby was born, and, from the way she looked at me, I knew that something wasn't right, but she didn't say anything at all. I remember telling her: "You need to talk to me, tell me what to do." And still—nothing. Then I asked: "What do you need me to do?" And then she finally asked me to take over for her. That was fine—I was the more experienced midwife, so we switched roles, and I took control of the situation. With the other new colleague, there was also a postpartum haemorrhage, but she had everything under control. She spoke clearly and directly, telling me what to do. We stayed in communication. That is absolutely essential when you work in a team. You have to know when to communicate verbally and when not. You can't freeze up.

(Team 2, focus group interview)

Verbal communication was the starting point for establishing effective communication, especially in emergency situations. However, during births, the experienced midwives emphasised the importance of quiet or non-verbal communication in order to preserve the calm atmosphere.

Reading non-verbal cues from new colleagues was especially difficult during the pandemic since the midwives wore FFP2 masks at births. One of the midwives in Team 1 explained:

Tilda: I've noticed, especially now with the masks, that it's even harder to read another person's facial expressions. Recently, I attended a birth with a new colleague, and she kept looking like this (makes a face: furrowing her brow). And I thought: Is she worried? Is something wrong? What's going on? Why does she keep looking at me like that? Am I doing something that she takes issue with? And then—(she laughs)—it actually turned out to be totally fine. The birth went well. Everything was okay. Afterward, I asked her what was going on with her and she said: "I think my forehead always looks like that. If I'm worried, I'll definitely say something out loud." And that was really reassuring for me to hear because the whole time I had been trying to read her eyes and was experiencing this weird internal feedback. But it made me realise again how much actually happens non-verbally between two midwives who are providing care together. And after the birth, we both said that, because she is new in the team, we really need to go outside occasionally and talk things through, so that we know that we're actually on the same page—otherwise, we might really misunderstand each other.

(Team 1, focus group interview)

In interpersonal communication studies, successful communication occurs when a message is intentionally or unintentionally sent and accurately decoded (Burgoon et al., 2011). Burgoon et al. distinguish eight non-verbal coding systems as means through which meaning is created, transmitted, perceived, and interpreted (2011, pp. 240–241). These include:

1 Kinesics: The use and interpretation of body movements, such as gestures, facial expressions, and posture, to communicate meaning.
2 Vocalics: Non-verbal aspects of the voice, including tone, pitch, volume, pauses, and other sounds like sighs or laughter, that affect how messages are received.
3 Physical appearance: How a person looks, including clothing, hairstyle, accessories, and physical features—all of which can influence first impressions and ongoing interactions.
4 Proxemics: The use of space in communication, such as how close or far people stand or sit in relation to one another, and what that signals about relationships or comfort.
5 Haptics: Communication through touch, including the type, location, and intensity of touch (e.g. a gentle pat on the shoulder versus a firm handshake).
6 Chronemics: How time is used and experienced in communication—for example, how long someone waits to respond, whether an interaction feels rushed or calm, and what that signals about respect or urgency.
7 Environment and artefacts: The arrangement and presence of objects, furniture, images, and other material elements in a space, which influence how people feel and behave in that environment.
8 Olfactics: The role of scent and smell in communication, including body odours, perfumes, or environmental smells that affect perception and interpersonal dynamics.

In clinical situations in the free-standing birth centres, experienced midwives stressed the ability to read gestures, since these can and do influence decision-making and team interaction. As Clifford Geertz (1973) illustrated through the example of a wink, the same physical gesture can carry very different meanings depending on context. While nursing and midwifery research acknowledges the importance of verbal and non-verbal interaction with patients, few studies explore how healthcare professionals communicate non-verbally with each other. This underexplored aspect of clinical practice warrants further study.

Team intelligence

Beyond individual skills and moment-to-moment communication, there is a broader question of how a team works as a collective. What makes a team function well in all situations, emergency and non-emergency? Suzanne Gordon (2012) has conducted extensive research into healthcare teams and their impact on patient safety. She emphasises the importance of situational awareness and group cognition, which includes understanding body language, tone, and gestures within healthcare teams. She refers to this as **team intelligence**. According to Gordon (2012, p. 219),

> Team intelligence … involves being aware not only of what skills and material people have mastered but also of what they don't understand but need to. It means making sure that people speak the same language, share the same goals, have clear expectations, are not subverted by unclarified assumptions, and help one another maintain situational awareness.

In addition to this, team intelligence requires team members to draw on the diverse strengths of their colleagues, enabling individuals to contribute through sharing knowledge and engaging in collaborative thinking. This capacity to work collectively towards common goals means that formal rank is subordinated to a shared commitment to mutual understanding and purpose. Each voice in the team is important for the provision of safe care and must be heard and considered. In the organisational structures of the free-standing birth centres, shared commitment to the work was encouraged and expected. The flat hierarchies that characterised these settings created conditions in which all of the newly qualified midwives felt their voices were heard and their contributions valued.

Enchantment, awe, and presence at births

Beyond communication techniques and team structures, there is also the matter of how midwives experience, make sense of, and choreograph births. For this, a hermeneutic phenomenological lens becomes useful. In Heideggerian (1926/2006) terms, newly qualified midwives, when they begin working at a free-standing birth centre, are *thrown* (*geworfen*) into situations that are unfamiliar to them. Julian Young (2000) offers a compelling description of Heidegger's concept of thrownness. He writes:

> A central concept in Being and Time—arguably the central concept—is "thrownness". So far as its definition is concerned, thrownness is a technical

term which identifies the fact that every person, as a person (Dasein), finds itself "already in" a cultural tradition which delimits both the range of actions which it makes sense to perform, and of those which it is valuable to perform.

(Young, 2012, p. 188)

Newly qualified midwives are thrown into their free-standing birth centre and encounter birth dynamics and rhythms that are, for the most part, new. Within this thrownness, a mood (*Stimmung*) arises. This mood is beyond a mere subjective feeling; it is a mode of disclosure that shapes how situations are first encountered (Smythe & Spence, 2023). As Heidegger (1926/2006) articulates through the concept of *Befindlichkeit*, often translated as situatedness or attunement, people always find themselves already within situations in which the world is meaningful or matters in particular ways (Smythe & Spence, 2023). In the free-standing birth centres, such moods may initially be felt as anxiety, uncertainty, or awe.

Being-with-others at births, which includes labouring women, birth companions, and colleagues, can be understood as a gathering in which the deeper meaning of birth can be revealed (Crowther, 2020). When working with their experienced colleagues, newly qualified midwives begin to attune to the significance of the gathering that had been concealed or hidden in their clinical training. They develop responsiveness that allows the underlying meaning of birth in this context to come into view, or into the clearing. As Smythe and Spence wrote:

Our attuning awakens us to our mood of interest, or boredom, or frustration, drawing us in or turning us away. Moods reveal "how we find ourselves"… "Attuning-to" picks up our mood and, in doing so, draws us back from the ontological experience of immersion to ontically examine and name [our emotion].

(Smythe & Spence, 2023, p. 23)

Susan Crowther (2020), drawing on Heidegger, elaborates that attunement is not simply a personal emotional state but a shared, pre-reflective condition that makes experience meaningful. It is through attunement that the deeper dimensions of birth become available to perception. In this sense, the newly qualified midwives adapt to the birth centre's protocols and pace at the same time that they take part in its atmosphere. Their moods shift as they become attuned to what birth *is* in this setting, for this woman, at this moment. Attunement is the condition for the kind of presence that experienced midwives recognise as meaningful, and for the trust that begins to form between colleagues.

In the focus group interviews, the experienced midwives were able to see and sense when newly qualified midwives were "present" in the birthing room based on the way they carried themselves. Negative emotional states, which are visible in a person's posture, signalled to the experienced midwives when a newly qualified midwife was not really "there." One of the midwives in Team 3 shared:

Amanda: Well, I tend to really notice the new midwife's posture. What is her posture when she is present at a birth? Is she slouched over, inwardly dozing off? I have difficulties with them when that's the case.

(Team 3, focus group interview)

While newly qualified midwives were seldom described as being slouched over, each of the experienced midwives could remember a midwifery student or new colleague who appeared bored or disinterested. Such signs of disengagement are generally regarded as incompatible with the practice of presence at births, which lies at the heart of care in both free-standing birth centres and at home births. Midwifery presence at births where one-to-one care is given may look as if the midwife is not doing anything at times; however, midwives use their senses (e.g., visual, auditory, tactile, and olfaction) to assess women throughout labour. Simply being *in* the room does not capture the essence of what it means to *be[ing]-with-other* in the birthing room, where expressing engagement may be so subtle that it is imperceptible. This has been described in midwifery literature as "watchful expectancy" (Adams, 1994) or more recently as "watchful attendance" (de Jonge et al., 2021).

Far more often, the experienced midwives could recall with particular warmth instances when a newly qualified midwife expressed genuine awe or joy during antenatal appointments and at births. These emotions were implicitly anticipated, marking them as a rite of passage into the shared values of the team.

Elena: I'm really amazed at how in awe so many of the new midwives are when they are fresh from their studies. There was a newly qualified midwife who made a huge impression on me. She was so amazed at how calm everything is here—no bright lights, no one shouting, no power pushing. Just calm. She was relieved, almost surprised, that we were friendly and treated her well. After a birth I had with her, she came out of the birthing room and said that we don't do any of the things here that she learned to do in the hospital. She saw that we were patient and didn't need to intervene, which made her nervous at first. We were patient and waited for the perineum to stretch—it's what we do here. When our client gave birth, she was amazed. She said: We don't need bright lights and oxytocin drips and hectic and stress. We can wait.

(Team 2, focus group interview)

Heart-warming moments included witnessing the growth and self-confidence of their new colleagues. As I sat in a circle with the midwives in one of the focus groups, the tone was joyful, almost playful, as the team shared positive stories with each other and with me. As is evident in the following interview, experienced midwives often needed evidence in a colleague's practical and relational skills before trusting them with more responsibility. One of the midwives said:

Tracy: I'm thinking of one new midwife in particular, Annika, who was so incredibly impatient at the beginning. Actually, almost all the new colleagues are like that. In any case, she wanted to do everything right away at the beginning and didn't understand how we worked. Sometimes we even had arguments because she thought the orientation period was too long. During the orientation period, the new colleagues have to see how we work before they take on responsibility. They can experience how all the midwives in the team work and can adopt ways of working that suit them. The work here is not something that a midwife invents on her own.

When I train others, I sometimes find it difficult not to intervene in what they're doing. For example, there was a shift where I was the second midwife and Annika was the first midwife. When the baby came, she frantically lifted it out of the water and put it on the woman's chest. She became terribly nervous and anxious when the child didn't cry the second she took it out of the water. I wanted to take over at that point. I thought it was a shame for the parents and for the baby. It could have been such a beautiful moment. And, actually, I'm happy to hand over to the new colleagues—BUT—I have to care for the woman first if I haven't worked much with the new midwife or if don't trust her yet. I have to first get a good sense of everything. There was a shift where Annika was the second midwife. I cared for the woman at the beginning. She was a fast first-time mom, and everything was going very well. After a while I asked Annika if she wanted to take over. She knew the woman well and the woman knew her. It was such a beautiful birth! She was lit up and glowing afterwards and that's what I love about the new colleagues, to be able to observe that. I get so much out of that—those are really special moments. I'm usually pragmatic and not emotional, but that is super special. I saw her glowing, and she came out of the room a couple of centimetres taller. She knows why she's working in the birth centre. This colleague, after she finished her orientation, told me that she now knows why she needed an orientation period (Team 7, focus group interview).

Trust was situated and contingent, dependent on how newly qualified midwives responded in real-time to the constantly evolving dynamics in the birth centre in general, and at births specifically. As Rocca-Ihenacho et al. (2021) observed in their study, a well-functioning midwifery unit depends on a positive work culture, where trust is actively fostered through shared practice, mutual respect, and psychological safety.

For experienced midwives, the emotional resonance, verbal clarity, and non-verbal responsiveness of the newly qualified midwives all signalled a growing alignment with the values of the team. Experienced midwives spoke of these moments with warmth, recognising them as turning points in individual development and affirmations of the shared work in the free-standing birth centre. In witnessing a colleague's awe, attentiveness, or appropriate action, experienced midwives saw their own practice reflected and renewed.

Questions for reflection

1 What subtle behaviours or moments help you determine whether a new colleague is beginning to arrive into your team, not just clinically, but relationally and culturally?
2 How do you personally balance the need to assess a new colleague's competence with fostering an atmosphere of trust, safety, and mutual respect?
3 Can you recall a time when your own communication, verbal or non-verbal, either supported or hindered collaboration during a birth? What did you learn from that moment?
4 How do you interpret the unspoken expectations in your team, and what helps you feel confident enough to ask for clarification or guidance when you are unsure?
5 When you reflect on your early experiences during births, what moments stand out as signals that you were beginning to be seen and trusted by your colleagues?
6 How do you notice and respond to the moods, gestures, or communication styles of the midwives you are learning from, and how is this shaping your own approach to being present with others during birth?

References

Adams, A. E. (1994). *Reproducing the Womb*. Cornell University Press.

Benoit, C., Davis-Floyd, R., van Teiglingen, E., Sandall, J., & Miller, J. F. (2001). Designing Midwives: A comparison of educational models. In R. DeVries, S. Wrede, E. van Teiglingen, & C. Benoit (Eds.), *Birth by Design* (pp. 139–165). Routledge.

Burgoon, J. K., Guerrero, L. K., & Manusov, V. (2011). Nonverbal signals. In M. L. Knapp & J. A. Daly (Eds.), *The Sage Handbook of Interpersonal Communication* (4th ed., pp. 239–282). Sage.

Crowther, S. (2020). *Joy at Birth: An Interpretive, Hermeneutic, Phenomenological Inquiry*. Routledge.

de Jonge, A., Dahlen, H., & Downe, S. (2021, Jun). 'Watchful attendance' during labour and birth. *Sex Reprod Healthc, 28*, 100617. https://doi.org/10.1016/j.srhc.2021.100617

Foucault, M. (1977). *Discipline and Punish: The Birth of the Prison* (1st American ed.). Pantheon Books.

Geertz, C. (1973). *The Interpretation of Cultures: Selected Essays*. BasicBooks, A Division of HarperCollins Publishers.

Gordon, S. (2012). On teams, teamwork, and team intelligence. In R. Koppel & S. Gordon (Eds.), *First, Do Less Harm: Confronting the Inconvenient Problems of Patient Safety* (pp. 196–220). ILR Press.

Heidegger, M. (1926/2006). *Sein und Zeit*. Max Niemeyer Verlag.

Labouvie, E. (2007). Alltagswissen - Körperwissen - Praxiswissen - Fachwissen zur Aneignung, Bewertungs- und Orientierungslogik von Wissenskulturen. *Ber Wissenschaftsgesch, 30*, 119–134. https://doi.org/10.1002/bewi.200701253

Lave, J., & Wenger, E. (1991). *Situated Learning: Legitimate Peripheral Participation*. Cambridge University Press.

Rocca-Ihenacho, L., Yuill, C., & McCourt, C. (2021, Mar). Relationships and trust: Two key pillars of a well-functioning freestanding midwifery unit. *Birth, 48*(1), 104–113. https://doi.org/10.1111/birt.12521

Smythe, L., & Spence, D. (2023). Nurturing a spirit of attuning-to. In S. Crowther & G. Thomson (Eds.), *Hermeneutic Phenomenology in Health and Social Care Research* (pp. 21–36). Routledge.

Surtees, R. (2008, Mar). 'Inductions of labour': On becoming an experienced midwifery practitioner in Aotearoa/New Zealand. *Nurs Inq, 15*(1), 11–20. https://doi.org/10.1111/j.1440-1800.2008.00392.x

Young, J. (2000). What is dwelling? The homelessness of modernity and the worlding of the world. In M. A. Wrathall & J. Malpas (Eds.), *Heidegger, Authenticity, and Modernity: Essays in Honor of Hubert L. Dreyfus, Volume 1* (Vol. 1, pp. 187–204). The MIT Press.

Young, N. (2012, Dec). An exploration of clinical decision-making among students and newly qualified midwives. *Midwifery, 28*(6), 824–830. https://doi.org/10.1016/j.midw.2011.09.012

9

"NOT A GOOD FIT"

The challenge to feel at home in team care

Introduction

In Chapter 8, we explored the lived experience of experienced midwives as they supported newly qualified midwives during their orientation. Rather than focusing solely on clinical competence, they emphasised the importance of relational trust. Orientation was revealed to be a social process, grounded in mutual responsiveness and a shared care dynamic. In this chapter, the story of Bianca will be told through her lived experience and that of her colleagues. After only six months, Bianca's team told her that they would not continue with her orientation, a situation that seemed to occur from time to time in the free-standing birth centres I visited during this study. While I knew of some of Bianca's difficulties, I was surprised at our third and final interview to learn of her team's decision.

Getting to know each other

Bianca, a newly qualified midwife, first contacted me by email, expressing interest in taking part in the study. At the time I met with her, I had already completed data collection with five newly qualified midwives in their first year of orientation and was comfortable with the recruitment process. We met for the first time on a warm autumn day at a farmer's market across town from the birth centre. She had just passed her final examinations and was looking forward to starting her first job as a midwife in a well-established free-standing birth centre. I picked her out right away in the crowd. She definitely had a midwife vibe. I told her about the study and what participation would involve, giving her ample opportunity to ask questions. After that, we chatted about this and that, taking time to get acquainted with each other. Our conversation was relaxed and friendly. I felt that we were able to build good

DOI: 10.4324/9781003591306-9

rapport in our first meeting, which boded well for the honest conversations I felt would surely follow. I was genuinely delighted that Bianca wanted to participate.

At her first interview several months later, we sat in her free-standing birth centre in one of the rooms used for antenatal appointments. She was bubbling over with enthusiasm as she told me stories from her first weeks of orientation. The conversation with Bianca that day was heartfelt. She told me about the first births she had observed and her relief at working with empathic midwives. She cried briefly when she spoke of the lack of empathy she had experienced from hospital midwives during her training in contrast to the warmth she now felt from her birth centre team, both towards their clients and towards her. She seemed uninhibited and joyful and was able to discuss clinical situations with ease.

Thrownness

Bianca, like the other newly qualified midwives in this study, found herself in Heideggerian (1962/2001) terms, thrown into a world not of her own making. In other words, Bianca entered a world that had long been established before her arrival. Even when chosen, these situations can feel unfamiliar, and we must find a way to dwell within them. We cannot choose that we are thrown, but we can face our thrownness. Bianca's stories, while deeply personal, also reflect the thrownness that the other newly qualified midwives experienced.

A helpful way to understand Heidegger's notion of thrownness is through a simple example. Imagine that ten people are brought to the edge of a wide, unfamiliar field early in the morning. Fog hangs in the damp, cold air, and the ground is riddled with molehills. The unevenness of the ground is enshrouded in mist, obscuring the contours of the small mounds. Each person is asked to walk across the field. While the field is the same for everyone, the experience of walking through it is not. They all enter the same field, but they do not encounter the same world.

Heidegger would say that this is not just about personality, mood, or consciousness. It concerns Dasein or "there-being" (Heidegger, 2017 in Rouse, 2013, p. 201), which he defines as the human way of existing as already embedded in a meaningful world (Wrathall, 2011). Dasein is not a subject inside a person, but the open space or clearing in which things show up as mattering. What someone notices or finds possible is shaped less by personal preferences than by how they are attuned in the world. This attunement is not emotional in the usual sense; it is ontological. It structures how the world appears as intelligible at all, revealing certain possibilities while obscuring others (Crowther et al., 2014). In this sense, the world is not simply encountered; it is disclosed. When someone begins to walk across the field, they are already situated in it in a particular way, even before conscious reflection begins. What is revealed differs for each person, depending on how the world is disclosed through their attunement.

This ontological insight becomes especially relevant when considering Bianca's early reflections. In her initial voice messages and at her first interview, Bianca told me about challenging situations at births. One of the first births she observed involved the transfer of a client with a previous caesarean section from the birth centre to a hospital. Her account of the situation leading to the transfer gave the appearance that she had sound clinical awareness and emotional composure. Nothing in her tone suggested uncertainty or distress. On the contrary, she seemed to be well adjusted. This is the voice message sent the day after the birth:

> Hi Nancy, I thought I'd send you a voice message today about a birth from yesterday. It was my first transfer. It wasn't an emergency, but also not something where we would transfer the woman by private car, so we called an ambulance. She had been at the birth centre all day, and I stayed the whole time, even after the shift change at 8pm. Throughout the day, she had regular contractions but also periods of rest where she slept. She was in the tub for an hour or so when we noticed that she had a slightly increased bloody show, even though she was fully dilated, so we got her out of the tub and moved to the mat in front of the bed. She had a reflexive urge to push and started pushing. During contractions, the baby's head would descend into the pelvic inlet but didn't really come any further down. When the fetal heart rate dropped slightly, we decided to transfer. She ended up having a vacuum extraction at the hospital—both mom and baby were great after the birth.
>
> I didn't think for a second that the situation was bad. I understood the whole time what was going on. From what I could see and hear in how my colleague spoke with our client, it was never stressful. Everything was communicated clearly and handled in a way that made me feel safe. I never felt afraid for the baby for even a moment. I really saw that my colleague transferred early rather than waiting for the situation to get urgent. I never once felt uncertain and was comfortable the whole time.
>
> *(Bianca, voice message 2)*

As a newly qualified midwife, encountering a situation like this at one of her first births could easily have been overwhelming. But in both her voice message and our interview, Bianca spoke with professional clarity. This left a strong, positive impression on me. The second birth she observed was no less complex, and again, in the way she described her experience, there was no hesitation or unease. Her accounts were vivid and grounded in detail, and she came across as someone with emotional depth. I would later realise that my perspective had been limited by a lack of contextual relationality between Bianca and her colleagues.

Unhomeliness *(Unheimlichkeit)*

By Bianca's second interview, some issues surfaced that she had expressed to me in a voice message sent shortly before our meeting. I could hear in her voice, which was a bit shaky and distressed, that she had been taken by surprise by the evaluation of her colleagues. In the voice message, she told me:

> I thought I'd tell you a bit more today about my orientation period. I have to say, in some situations I feel very unsure of myself, but I've done my first antenatal appointments on my own, and I've become more confident. What I really wanted to tell you about was the talk I had with my mentors and another colleague yesterday. At my first feedback session with them, I hadn't had many appointments or births yet. It was all pretty superficial. But at the feedback session yesterday, well—it wasn't quite as positive and certainly not what I had hoped for. I've always known about myself that I'm super reserved when I start something new. That's just how I've always been. Well, it came up in my mentors' feedback. They actually asked whether I really want to work at the birth centre as part of the team. That really hurt, that it came across as if I wasn't taking things seriously, or that I didn't really want to work there.
>
> It wasn't all criticism or doubt—there was a lot of encouragement too. They said they believe I can do the work, that they're sure I know what I'm doing, but it's like I don't have the courage to assert myself. They said that when other colleagues are in the room, I hold back too much. So, we tried to find some strategies to make it easier for me. At times I've felt really discouraged, and I doubt myself—even over small things. Yeah. I'm very hard on myself and have very high expectations. It's definitely a lot of new stuff all at once, and sometimes I really do feel like I'm hitting my limits. I definitely notice that.
>
> *(Bianca, voice message 3)*

This message was the first sign I received from Bianca that she was not feeling at home in her team. She had yet to experience a sense of arrival. She felt misunderstood, while, at the same time, feeling grateful that her colleagues wanted to help her overcome her timidity. She was convinced that she wanted to stay, but something had shifted. She was feeling as if the world she had been thrown into was no longer reassuring.

In Heideggerian terms, she was moving into a state of unhomeliness (*Unheimlichkeit*), also translated as uncanniness (Withy, 2013). According to Heidegger (1971), this is not merely a feeling; it is a basic trait of human existence. Bianca experienced an existential disruption in the way the world showed up for her and in the way she was showing up for her team. Where she had once been open and motivated, she now felt disconnected and dislocated. The familiarity with her colleagues that she spoke of in her first interview had given way to an unsettling distance. She was still in the world of the birth centre but could no longer dwell in it easily. Bianca said this in her second interview:

> I was caring for a labouring woman with another colleague, who was offering care with me. She asked me if it would be okay if she stepped back a little and I

did more of the care – as the primary midwife. I thought it would be a bit easier for me that way. Like I told you in that voice message – it's always been hard for me when someone else is present with me, but it depends, I guess. With some, I feel under pressure, and with others not at all.

(Bianca, second interview)

Bianca's experience was not simply one of failing to fit in; it revealed a more fundamental reality: that being at home in the world is never settled. It is always shaped by the way we find ourselves situated in it. Heidegger (1926/2006) wrote that the state of not feeling at home is not just a disruption or a temporary break-down; it is a more fundamental way of being. This does not mean that we are always anxious, but that the sense of homeliness we rely on in our everyday lives is itself a mode of something deeper, an underlying uncanniness that is part of what it means to be human. Bianca, as much as she loved being a midwife, did not feel at home being-with her colleagues in the room, which was a distinguishing feature of working in her free-standing birth centre and foundational to the team's concept of safe care.

Bianca's situation in her free-standing birth centre quickly became more tenuous. I was interested in understanding her team's perspective, so I spent a few days in observation at the birth centre. During a four-day rapid ethnography session, I was able to talk to several midwives in the team. Here is an excerpt from one of our recorded conversations:

I had three or four births with Bianca that were all very straightforward, where the women simply came and gave birth. There was no need for an interven-tion, and there were no emergencies. But, especially at the water birth we had together, she wasn't able to communicate with the woman. It was if she wasn't really present for us. I had even explained to her in detail what she needed to do, since she didn't have any experience with water birth in her clinical prac-tice. She not only didn't do what we had discussed; she did nothing—she said nothing and didn't proceed how we had discussed beforehand. In the team, we all get the feeling that when we're with her at a birth that she doesn't dare to be present, let alone take the lead. She fades away and waits for us to do everything. When we've talked about it afterwards with her, we weren't even sure that she was understanding what we meant. One of the colleagues who worked with her asked her beforehand if she felt confident enough to be the second midwife at a birth. She said yes. When a client began to bleed postpar-tum, she seemed to overlook it, even though the colleague was signalling to her that she needed assistance. Instead of acting appropriately, she stroked the woman's arm. We've gone through emergency scenarios with her, so we know that she knows where everything is and knows what to do, but she enters into a zone where we can't seem to reach her. We just don't know: does she see the situation and can't assess it properly? Does she not see it at all for what it is? Or does she see it and is too afraid to communicate with us and carry out what needs to be done? The really hard part is that we keep asking her to tell us what she sees. We can't let her work on her own if she can't communicate and act appropriately in urgent situations. And I think very often she simply doesn't notice it. That isn't a reason during orientation to ask a colleague to leave. It's not problematic, if I can give someone feedback afterward and say, hey, I noticed this or that. But when we ask her afterwards, we can't tell whether she truly saw what was happening and froze – or didn't see it at all and only says she did. We're left not knowing what's real for her in those moments, and we need her to see things how we see them—as they ARE. There are situations – reality – that cannot be negotiated.

(Rapid ethnography 5)

During my observation period at the free-standing birth centre, Bianca was told that the team could no longer carry her through orientation. There had been a time in the past when they had invested more time and effort into a colleague who needed a longer orientation, but Bianca's lack of palpable presence at births left the team feeling that she needed a more structured, clinical environment as a newly qualified midwife.

Das Man: 'The they' and discourse

What emerged in the team's reflections was not simply that Bianca struggled with communication or fitting into team norms, but that her presence was marked by a kind of absence. She was there, yet not in a way that was meaningful to them. Bianca described herself in the following way:

Sometimes I find it difficult when I'm the second midwife – and someone else is the first midwife – because the first midwife often takes up so much space that I don't really know what I'm supposed to do. Maybe it's not that I physically withdraw, but I'm not the kind of person who enters a room and radiates a lot of dominance. I tend to adapt and subordinate myself.

(Bianca, third interview)

Heidegger (1926/2006) writes that we typically navigate the world through the shared, impersonal expectations of *das Man*, the anonymous 'the they,' where appropriate behaviour is taken-for-granted; and things are done how they have always been done. Hence, 'the they' is a mode of being characterised by conformity and everydayness (Wrathall, 2011). While Heidegger associates it with inauthenticity, he does not present it as inherently negative. On the contrary, it enables us to function within a shared world, moving fluidly through familiar practices and routines. In a free-standing birth centre, or any clinical environment, this taken-for-granted structure is essential. It provides the baseline orientation for action, not necessarily by way of personal deliberation, but by doing what 'one does' in any particular situation. For Bianca, not entering into this mode of shared understanding left her team unsure whether she could be counted on to respond appropriately in emergency situations. They expected her to offer care with the colleague she was working with, as opposed to being subordinate to them.

Being-with colleagues: Offering collaborative care

In Bianca's free-standing birth centre, antenatal care was structured around collaborative, shared care. Orientation was not conceived as a test, but as opportunities for being-with, where mutual and interactive understanding could take shape. The hope was that through this process, the newly qualified midwife would gradually get integrated into the team. However, Bianca experienced these moments as implicitly evaluative rather than shared. She told me:

> I feel like those [appointments], when I'm alone with a client, well, they're just completely different from when we're in pairs. I feel so much better than when, for example, another midwife is with me, but I'm the one doing most of the talking. I don't have that many appointments on my own yet—some aren't even scheduled—so I still go with the other midwives, or we alternate a bit. And in those shared appointments, I find it much harder because the midwife is always so quiet and just expects me to lead the conversation. When I'm alone I know that no one will judge or evaluate what I say. Those conversations are much more relaxed and also much nicer for me.
>
> *(Bianca, second interview)*

The feedback Bianca received may have reflected something deeper: that her responses had not yet aligned with the shared practices of the team. Her developing identity as a birth centre midwife remained concealed. Bianca had become ontologically dislocated and alone, in spite of feeling that she was capable of connection.

While the team increasingly perceived Bianca's presence as unreadable or even unsafe, her own descriptions of care, marked by empathy and meticulousness, tell a parallel story. These two narratives do not cancel each other out. Rather, they circle the same experience from different vantage points, revealing the fragility of being-with in a space where both spoken and embodied communication were essential. Bianca had completed her midwifery training, passed her exams, and entered the free-standing birth centre with the same qualifications as her peers. In our conversations, she came across as empathic, reflective, and articulate. I did not experience her as emotionally distant or unreliable. Yet the team's unease was persistent and, ultimately, decisive. They described moments, particularly during births, when her actions were difficult to read, or her responses were out of sync with what the situation required.

This presents a dialectic worth holding open: Bianca's being-in-the-world made sense in the context of our conversations, where her reflections were clear and clinically grounded, but in the world of the birth centre, her knowledge remained hidden. While I did not understand this as a failure of her training, it served as a reminder to me that being-with in the free-standing birth centres required an adjustment period to adapt and broaden skills for working in a particular team.

Bianca's journey felt awkward and posed a challenge for me when I reflected on her interviews in light of what her team had shared with me, since I had truly treasured our time together. However, in a free-standing birth centre, teamwork is fundamental to safe care. Midwives act side-by-side, often wordlessly, relying on one another to notice, respond, and adjust in real time. Bianca's colleagues did not doubt her good intentions, but they described her as unreadable in moments that called for spontaneous coordination. Her presence, though calm and reflective in the interviews, did not translate into the attuned engagement required in everyday clinical practice. Her team's decision to end her orientation was a recognition of the specific demands of the setting. Skill acquisition takes time and extends beyond the formal orientation period, and no one is expected to know everything from the start. However, according to this team, the ability to work collaboratively is essential to providing safe care. In one of the focus group interviews, an experienced midwife said that their team motto was: *Together we are genius*, recognising the significance of input from each member of the team, even the least experienced, and underscoring that safe care emerges only when each voice finds its place in the whole.

Questions for reflection

1 What have your experiences been like working within a midwifery team?
2 When have you felt a sense of belonging? When have you felt "dislocated," as if you do not belong?
3 Do you think every midwife can feel at home in any team setting? Why or why not?
4 What kinds of practices or interactions can foster a sense of ease, trust, and mutual understanding in a newly qualified midwife?
5 Beyond clinical competence, what helps someone genuinely participate in shared care and be-with others in meaningful ways?

References

Crowther, S., Smythe, L., & Spence, D. (2014, Mar). Mood and birth experience. *Women Birth, 27*(1), 21–25. https://doi.org/10.1016/j.wombi.2013.02.004
Heidegger, M. (1926/2006). *Sein und Zeit*. Max Niemeyer Verlag.
Heidegger, M. (1962/2001). *Being and Time* (J. Macquarrie & E. S. Robinson, Trans.; 7th ed.). Blackwell Publishers.

Heidegger, M. (1971). *Poetry, Language, Thought* (1st ed.). Harper & Row.
Rouse, J. (2013). Dasein. In M. A. Wrathall (Ed.), *The Cambridge Companion to Heidegger's Being and Time* (pp. xx, 426). Cambridge University Press.
Withy, K. (2013). Uncanniness. In M. A. Wrathall (Ed.), *The Cambridge Companion to Heidegger's Being and Time* (pp. xx, 426). Cambridge University Press.
Wrathall, M. A. (2011). *Heidegger and Unconcealment: Truth, Language, and History.* Cambridge University Press.

10

"SHE WAS LABOURING IN A RAIN BARREL WHEN WE ARRIVED!"

The surprising and awe-inspiring experiences of newly qualified midwives

Introduction

In Chapter 9, we followed Bianca's story, tracing how her inability to work well with her team ultimately led to the end of her contract with her free-standing birth centre. Despite her emotional depth, Bianca's presence did not translate into the kind of relational responsiveness her team expected. In this chapter, we explore the surprising and unforgettable moments that left a lasting impression on newly qualified midwives. These stories reveal how unexpected events can disrupt and move newly qualified midwives, leading to realisations that help them define their midwifery practice.

Stories that grip us: Stories worth telling

What moves, surprises, or disturbs newly qualified midwives? What grasps them so powerfully that their experience becomes a story to be told? In the newly qualified midwives' interviews, as well as in voice messages they left after particularly moving experiences, I was invited through their storytelling into moments that had stirred, awakened, or disturbed something within them. From the beginning of data collection, I was struck by the detail and depth of these stories, many of which moved me as well. The word *moving* comes from the Latin *movere*, meaning to set in motion or disturb, with roots in the Proto-Indo-European *meue*: to push away (Harper, n.d.). Being moved can draw us closer to people, places, and things, or push us away from them.

Some stories seem absurd or extraordinary and need to be told over and over, while others are subtle, yet powerful enough to initiate change. They can repel us, as the root *meue* suggests, or fascinate us, prompting a shift in how we understand

DOI: 10.4324/9781003591306-10

the world. Deeply personal, midwifery stories often depict moments that are shaped through shared and relational practice. These are stories that endure and are worth retelling because they recall moments that caught us off guard and brought the world into sharper focus.

The phenomenologist Bernhard Waldenfels (2020) writes that feeling moved or disrupted when we are struck deeply by a person, situation, or event evokes a response before we consciously think things through. In this sense, the irritation or sudden feeling of being moved often feels like something that happens to "me," rather than something that "I" did (Waldenfels, 2004). We feel addressed, affected, or stung by an *other* or by a situation. The person or situation seems to demand a response, and, in our response, we often call on familiar norms or frameworks, referred to by Waldenfels as 'orders,' to find meaning (Schnegg, 2024). Waldenfels (2020, p. 353) writes that *We are unable to create and to invent **what** we are responding **to**, yet we do really have to invent and to create **what** we respond, making use of a sort of responsive creativity.* As a phenomenologist, Waldenfels did not believe that we construct reality, nor that we intentionally frame it, but that we have an inner response or an inner feeling of being moved before reflection takes place.

In everyday life, most experiences do not evoke a sense of an *other* or of something alien. We do not have to question those around us or our experiences with them, nor do we have an impulse to initiate change (Schnegg, 2024). However, in situations where there is a breakdown, what Heidegger calls unready-to-hand, we are called to respond creatively, since responsivity cannot be fixed or determined without risking a loss of openness to the *other* (Waldenfels, 2020, p. 353). When responsivity becomes rule-bound, a person, situation, or event may still address us, but the encounter is reduced to a functional exchange. In such moments, what might have disrupted our understanding and initiated change is overridden by rules or guidelines that value control over openness to the other. The stories shared below reflect these moments in which the newly qualified midwives were moved or disrupted from the familiar in response to people (clients and colleagues), situations, and events. Getting insight into their reflections shows pathways of growth, development, and boundary making.

Stepping into the unfamiliar

Felicia, a newly qualified midwife, left me a voice message with the following story, which she later retold during her interview. In both instances, the sound of her voice captivated me with its urgency. In the message, she sounded clearly rattled. As a midwife myself, I could vividly imagine how I might have reacted in her place. I was gripped by the disorientation, humour, and resolve woven through her account. This is her story of a birth in a rain barrel:

I want to tell you about a really outrageous situation at a birth. A woman was registered to give birth at the birth centre, however when she called with contractions, it was clear she wouldn't make it to us in time. So, we drove to her home—about 50 minutes away. I was officially the second midwife but had already been taking on first midwife responsibilities. I might have led this birth, too, if it hadn't been for the absurd situation we found ourselves in when we arrived. When we got there, we entered their apartment with our equipment and were led to the bathroom, which was in the farthest corner. It was a very, very, very small bathroom, really cramped, with a rain barrel in the very farthest corner—first the sink, and then in the corner in the shower stall: a rain barrel! Our client was labouring in a tall rain barrel. I couldn't even fit in the bathroom with the others, so I sat in the open bathroom door.

I saw clearly that my colleague got a grip on the situation quickly and also saw that she had no way to help the woman fish her baby out of the water after giving birth unless she entered the rain barrel with her. So, she told her: "I can't do anything if you have your baby in there—you'll have to lift it out yourself. I can't do anything." It was an absurd moment of total helplessness. Because of this, I am not a fan of rain barrels. It was very uncool.

I took on the task of documenting the birth. I had wanted to step into the lead, but my colleague already knew the woman—and frankly, I was taken aback by the rain barrel. I usually listen to the fetal heartbeats, but, like I said, I couldn't physically enter the room, so my colleague listened. She literally had to dive into the rain barrel to listen to them, which was the first thing she did when we arrived—the heartbeats were fine. Our client gave birth soon after.

The water wasn't even warm. We didn't want the baby getting hypothermia, so we got the woman out of the barrel right after the birth, even though she wanted to stay in longer. That was a real effort—she wasn't petite—and with the way the room was set up, it was nearly impossible. After this birth, the team met and reviewed the liability. We decided that we would no longer accept clients who planned to give birth in rain barrels.

(Felicia, first interview and voice message 1)

For Felicia, this situation was a lived disruption of her embodied, practiced way of being-with a woman in labour, triggering a feeling of estrangement. Nothing in her clinical training or orientation period had prepared her for this situation: a woman immersed up to her chest in a rain barrel, in the farthest corner of a cramped, inaccessible bathroom. There was no room for her to enter, no possibility to kneel beside the birthing woman, and no space to listen to fetal heartbeats without, as she put it, "diving in." The familiarity of performing second-midwife tasks, such as witnessing, monitoring, and preparing for the birth, was suddenly absent. Everything that formed a coherent world of birth assistance for her was spatially and practically unattainable.

Waldenfels (2004, p. 244) writes that

we are touched by others before being able to ask who they are and what their behaviour or their utterances mean. The other's otherness, which overcomes and surprises us, disturbs our intentions before being understood in this or that sense.

Felicia's experiential grounding was disrupted in ways that she could not quickly compensate for. While she was learning relational care in her orientation, she still relied on situations that were structurally familiar and stable. Her immediate response to the woman in the rain barrel did not lead to a creative solution, but to a boundary.

Quintessential calmness

While moments that disturb us may force a realisation in their urgency, tumbling into an unexpected situation can also engender admiration and awe. In this next story, what gripped the newly qualified midwife, Theresa, was not a dramatic disturbance but nevertheless a disturbance in how she had come to expect midwives to look and behave at births. She was struck by the utter repose of her colleague, whose way of being-with carried an effortless certainty. The moment stayed with her as a lived embodiment of poise. She told me:

> I was already on the schedule as the second midwife and was called by my colleague to come to a birth. So, of course, I raced down the highway to get here and pretended to arrive all casual, as if my heart wasn't beating like a rabbit from the drive. The birth centre wasn't well lit when I walked in, and my colleague was just sitting there at the front table with the client file and papers stacked neatly in front of her, knitting and drinking tea. The couple was in one of the birthing rooms when I arrived—I could hear that the woman was already fairly far along, vocal toning loudly during the contractions. I was awe-struck. My colleague was seriously—no joke—just sitting there knitting. I asked her: "Huh? What's up?" And she said casually: "Oh hi." And I asked: "Did I miss something?" And she said: "No, no, they wanted to be alone for a moment."
>
> The other births I had been at before this one were with other colleagues. Each colleague had her own way of caring for labouring women, and this colleague was somehow completely different from them. She was so relaxed! She was actually wearing all white, from head to toe. I immediately thought: Wow, she's so composed. The fact that she was so calm, wearing white—but, you know—the births here are always "clean"—which might sound strange. They're not at all like the births I attended in the hospital, which always seemed so bloody. I immediately thought: I'll do that someday, too. One day I'll also wear all white, and one day this will all just flow for me. Yeah, it was kind of crazy. I don't know, it just—it stuck with me.
>
> *(Theresa, first interview)*

What Theresa witnessed was not dramatic, yet it oriented her to a new way of being. The contrast between her quickly beating heart and her colleague's composure caught her off guard. Heidegger (1954) writes that what is most thought-provoking is often what is most unassuming. The midwife's relaxed posture, the knitting, and her white clothing were for Theresa both ordinary and exemplary. For Waldenfels

(2020), the turn from being moved or touched to responding is central to how we become who we are. Theresa experienced a way of being that was not yet her own, but something she could turn towards and cultivate.

A shift in being-with: Transforming risk perceptions

The newly qualified midwife Sally also experienced a shift that transpired quietly, albeit deeply. She suddenly became aware of how she regarded birth before starting at the birth centre and how this had shifted after several months, setting off a chain reaction in her thinking. She said:

> Yesterday I was at a birth that was totally physiological—no interventions. The more I witness, the more I am able to let go of my fears. These aren't conscious fears that I've brought with me. There is something deeper, where I'm beginning to realise that it is possible to have confidence in the birth process, which feels really good. Then, on Tuesday, I had a meeting with my first actual client, a woman whom I will accompany throughout her entire pregnancy. Her due date is in June, when I'll finally be on-call as the primary midwife at births. And I noticed during the course of the conversation how strongly I am still caught up in the mindset of "what can go wrong?"
>
> And then at some point, a switch flipped, and I could suddenly feel that beautiful sense of what it means for me to work at the birth centre. I don't know how that happened. I suddenly realised while I was talking to her that I was actually just telling her what it is we do here at the birth centre—what our routine is, and it suddenly dawned on me: of course! We provide one-to-one care and have a really rigorous selection process. Complications here are so rare. I noticed how much I still needed to let go of. It's still really tied up with my time in the hospital—where we experienced complications all the time and constantly had to prepare for them. But now, I'm watching women simply give birth. They can do it! They can manage! There are really beautiful births here. I guess it will get better with every positive experience I have. Deciding to come work at the birth centre means a huge change for me in my very being—I can feel that—that even my character, everything about who I am—is changing. I'm finally calming down a bit. I can feel how tense I've been. I was at so many births this past week, along with postnatal visits during the day. I'm completely wired. I might even be feeling a bit lost, but I think that's because I'm going through such a huge change. So, my takeaway from what I just told you is: Letting go so that the change I'm going through can just be. Then I can arrive and relax and accept who I am becoming.

(Sally, voice message 11)

Sally's encounters with beautiful births clashed with her learned and familiar positioning from hospital births, shifting her understanding. Having been trained to respond to labouring women with attention to what could go wrong, she felt both freed and disoriented at the same time, finally able to let go of her anxiety. Sally neither consciously chose the situations that affected her, nor could she have engineered her transformation. She was touched by situations and events that unsettled her familiar orientation and did more than just change her mind; it shifted her responsiveness to labouring and birthing women, as well as to the birth centre itself.

Witnessing wisdom: Revealing the significance of relationship dynamics

Nanette recounted witnessing something entirely new to her at a home birth in her orientation period. What unfolded offered her a new perspective on how emotional entanglements can surreptitiously shape the course of birth, revealing how birth progresses when inner and outer readiness align. Reflecting on the experience, Nanette described it this way:

> I was at a birth of a client recently who I'm still visiting postnatally. I have to admit, I was still so nervous and was very happy that all I was supposed to do was document the birth because I didn't really know what to do, and I still love just observing. It was our client's third birth, and, in spite of the fact that her kids were at home and had to get ready for school, she was totally relaxed. The kids had to be ready for school by 6 a.m., which meant getting them sorted and out the door. Her mother arrived to help out, but she was still saying things between contractions like, "Mom, you still need to pack the lunchboxes," and "The backpacks are right here." She was completely preoccupied with getting the kids ready and out the door—even though she could have left all that to her mother. It didn't feel off to me, how she was. On the contrary, I thought it was impressive that she still had the mental space to think about her kids in the middle of labour—and was even helping get everything ready for them. It was remarkable that she could do all that while still managing her contractions, which were really strong—and she just took it all in stride. I was there with two colleagues. One told me: "She can't let go. She's still caught up with her kids. Once they're gone, she'll have the baby quickly." I didn't really see this—like, I didn't get it. I guess, for my colleagues, it was predictable, but not for me. And that's exactly what happened. Before her daughter left with Grandma, she came in for a moment, gave her mom a kiss on the forehead, and then went off to school. That moment was so emotional—and maybe it's exactly what she needed: to know that the kids were okay with everything. And then she could finally let go. She gave birth quickly after that. It was a beautiful birth and a great experience for me.
>
> *(Nanette, first interview)*

For newly qualified midwives who have completed their clinical training in environments where the birth dynamic was often concealed by interventions, their orientation in a free-standing birth centre and at home births may be the first time they encounter this kind of birth dynamic. In addition to gaining a sense of how birth unfolds when left largely undisturbed, they must also learn to navigate the complex presence of others at birth. This includes the birth companion, and sometimes children, extended family, or friends. Unlike the more controlled and hierarchical setting of the hospital, where presence is often peripheral and managed, free-standing birth centres and home births welcome a broader, more participatory constellation of relationships. Newly qualified midwives must learn to perceive how these shifting dynamics affect both the birthing woman and them. At the heart of this is learning that birth does not need to be managed, merely because it is complex. In free-standing birth centres and at home births, dynamics are observed and responded to as they evolve and shift.

She sucked on my finger!: Re-orienting after the unexpected

Vaginal examinations are conducted by midwives to discern cervical dilation, fetal position, and fetal station. Yet they are never a neutral act, in spite of being routinised. Conducted in the shared space of embodied presence, the encounter includes not only the labouring woman but also the fetus, which may, at times, respond to touch, moving and even rotating their head. The following account describes such a moment, when Amelia was confronted with something entirely unexpected during what she anticipated would be a routine examination.

> So, my very first birth alone was during the night in the birth centre. Um, yeah, at some point I did a vaginal examination—she was in the tub—and I was totally taken off guard—actually, shocked—because, you only ever expect to feel the head, but what I felt reacted to my touch: it wrinkled its nose, squinted its eyes, and sucked on my finger. Wild! And then I thought, oh fu(dge). I quickly went through the list in my head, like: the heartbeats are good. Where is the back of the baby? Is it in the right position for a vaginal birth? I was honestly so surprised when the baby started to suck on my finger but of course had to stay calm. I called my second midwife right away, mostly because our client was giving birth to her second baby, and the head was already descending into the birth canal. I asked her to get out of the tub and was very firm about it. I didn't have much experience with water births and zero experience with face presentation. As she was getting out, my second midwife arrived. Shortly after that, we could see the mouth and the nose at the pelvic floor. It was a really fast birth—the baby was born a half hour after the vaginal exam.
>
> *(Amelia, third interview)*

Amelia's response to the baby sucking on her finger was a shock from which she quickly recovered, using a clinical framework to understand the situation and guide her responsivity. For her this meant asking her client to get out of the bathtub, an understandable boundary for a midwife leading her first birth. Rather than being a fixed boundary, it emerged from the situation itself, as Amelia requested what she needed to provide care within her skill-set. Despite her excitement, she remained calm in the face of a strange and unexpected moment. She was able to continue giving care after her assessment, and, in doing so, she remained open to the extraordinary.

The stories in this chapter have traced moments in which newly qualified midwives were gripped by the unexpected. Each surprise and disruption clearly display an emotional response followed by a confrontation with an ideal, a way of relating, or a routine. Their stories show how clinical learning includes being affected, disturbed, and compelled to change, bringing forth new ways of seeing, understanding, and responding, as well as prompting boundary making.

Questions for reflection

1 Have you ever been surprised, moved, or unsettled by something during clinical practice? What made that moment stay with you?
2 What kinds of experiences leave a lasting impression on you? Why?
3 How do moments of surprise or disruption shape your understanding of what it means to be a midwife?
4 Can being "seized" by an experience (emotionally, ethically, bodily) help us grow in our practice? How?
5 What helps you stay open and responsive when a birth doesn't unfold the way you expected?

References

Harper, D. (n.d.). *Move*. https://www.etymonline.com/word/move
Heidegger, M. (1954). *Was Heisst Denken?* M. Niemeyer.
Schnegg, M. (2024). Cutlure as response. *Ethos, 52*(2), 308–323. https://doi.org/10.1111/etho.12427
Waldenfels, B. (2004). Bodily experience between selfhood and otherness. *Phenomenol Cogn Sci, 3*, 235–248. https://doi.org/10.1023/B:PHEN.0000049305.92374.0b
Waldenfels, B. (2020). Responsivity and co-responsivity from a phenomenological point of view. *Stud Phænomenologica, XX*, 341–355. https://doi.org/10.5840/studphaen20202015

11

"I WAS THE LAST MIDWIFE TO HEAR THE FETAL HEARTBEATS." INTRAUTERINE DEATH IN MIDWIFERY PRACTICE

Introduction

In Chapter 10, we turned our attention to the awe-inspiring and disorienting moments that gripped newly qualified midwives, illuminating how unexpected experiences, ranging from births in rain barrels to subtle shifts in perception, can shape a midwife's becoming. These stories underscored the transformative power of being seized by the moment, revealing how midwives grow through surprise, reflection, and presence. In this chapter, we turn to one of the most profound and sorrowful realities of midwifery practice: stillbirth. I will explore intrauterine death before the onset of labour, and how midwives come to dwell with grief, not only their own, but also the grief of others. Through narrative, reflection, and poetry, I examine how such experiences carve themselves into the heart of practice and how, even in the absence of life, midwives need to remain present, attentive, and human.

"Invisible death": Stillbirth

This chapter will focus on stillbirth, specifically on intrauterine death before the onset of contractions, which has been described as "invisible death" (Defrain, 1986 in Cacciatore & Bushfield, 2007). The tragedy of death when life should begin marks parents with an indescribable grief that endures (Burden et al., 2016; Cacciatore & Bushfield, 2007). As midwives, we are not outside the sphere of grief at stillbirths (Kenworthy & Kirkham, 2011). The sorrow we feel is not the same as that of the parents, but it is real. It lives within us in its own way, moving differently through us than through the family. It is shaped by the responsibility we carry, the intimacy of the care we give, and the compassion and heartache that we share when a pregnancy does not end as expected. In German, there is a

DOI: 10.4324/9781003591306-11

word—*Weltschmerz*—that gestures towards this kind of pain. It describes a deep sensitivity to suffering in the world, and the emotional weight one may carry in response to it, even when the loss is not one's own. For many midwives, this quiet, enduring sorrow becomes part of their internal landscape. In this chapter, I will be sharing my own experiences as a midwife caring for women during labour who knew that their baby would not take its first breath. I will also, through poetry, share the story of a newly qualified midwife who was the last person to hear the heartbeats of a baby at a house visit during the night.

Hardships in midwifery practice

When people ask me about my work, they are asking about live births, enthusiastic about hearing the ins and outs of such a special profession. They imagine that experiencing birth on a regular basis is thrilling and joyful. Since I am not cynical at heart, I usually nod, and, only on rare occasions tell them that I wish that would be the case, but, no, actually there are, from time to time, very difficult days in midwifery practice. It is not the frequency of these days that defines their weight, but the way their possibility shapes how we work, how we speak, and how we perceive labour and birth (Scamell, 2011). Among those difficult days, the ones involving unexpected loss have stayed with me the longest.

Although intrauterine death at term is statistically rare in most high-income countries, the spectre of it looms large. Jo Murphy-Lawless has argued that the risk discourse underpins obstetric care during pregnancy and instrumentalises this fear, not because death is common, but because its possibility wields power (1998). In Heideggerian (1962/2001) terms, this fear reflects our unease in the face of Being-towards-death (*Sein-zum-Tode*), an ontological condition that modern obstetrics often tries to mask through control and surveillance. Yet even in its rarity, the idea of death shapes behaviour, policy, and emotion. It haunts not because it is probable, but because it is irreversible, and because it breaks the expected arc of birth as pure beginning. However, the fantasy that with sufficient technology, surveillance, and the proper diet and behaviour, babies will not die in utero or in the neonatal period has simply not come to be (Lupton, 2012; Murphy-Lawless, 1998; Thompson, 2012).

As a newly qualified midwife, I did not begin practising midwifery naively. I had witnessed fetal loss during my clinical training, situations that rendered me speechless for days. At the time of my training, the policy in the hospital was to immediately remove stillborn babies from their parents. The belief was that the sight of the baby would be agonising and trauma inducing for the parents (Komaromy, 2012). Those experiences left me with many unresolved issues. Accordingly, I promised myself that I would engage differently with families experiencing stillbirth when I became a midwife. Although my dream had been to be a home birth midwife or to work in a free-standing birth centre, something that carried personal meaning for me from the beginning, in my first ten years practising midwifery,

I worked in two different hospital labour wards. In the second hospital, I worked in a magnificent team with very experienced midwives and enjoyed work on most days. The shifts that were most demanding were those where I supported families navigating complex social, emotional, or economic hardships, as well as loss.

Over the years, I cared for women who, during an antenatal appointment, either a routine CTG or ultrasound, were told that their baby's heart was no longer beating. Most often, we would receive a phone call from an obstetric physician's practice informing us that they were sending over a woman whose baby had died. Those were moments where we all held our breath and prepared for grief. We midwives would speak amongst ourselves to check in and decide who felt emotionally equipped to offer care. We found it important when providing care in these situations to be able to dwell with pain and grief. When possible, we made sure that the midwife offering care was not simultaneously supporting a woman labouring with a live child, and when feasible, we tried to avoid a shift change so that the woman wouldn't have to get accustomed to a new midwife—something we could unfortunately not always achieve. It was rare at that hospital that we discovered the fetal death ourselves. Usually, the women arrived with a diagnosis. Several years in a row, I happened to be on shift each time a woman arrived with a stillborn baby, and each time, I cared for her.

Connection, grief, miracle

Many years ago, at the beginning of one of my late shifts, the bell rang in the labour and delivery ward, signalling that a patient was at the door. The labour and delivery ward housed both the gynaecology and obstetrics departments, so that we never knew when we went to the door to receive people if we would greet a pregnant woman or a gynaecological patient. On this day, a couple in their mid-30s was standing at the door, both of them crying. The woman was holding her belly, trembling. Both had reddened eyes, and, when I caught the woman's gaze, her grief seemed to widen and draw me in. What had been a private moment for them up until then was now shared. My presence, even before a single word was spoken, made what had been unspeakable now unbearably real. She reached for me, unable to carry the weight of her anguish alone, and I opened my arms to hold her. I then guided them to a quiet room, separate from the usual birthing rooms.

Alone with the couple in a home-like room, they told me that they had been to her obstetrician for a routine antenatal check. When the fetal heartbeats could not be detected using the fetal heart monitor, her obstetrician performed an ultrasound and confirmed that the baby's heart had stopped beating. Disoriented and overwhelmed, the couple came straight to us—to the hospital where she had given birth to her other children. After listening to her story, the attending physician performed a confirmatory scan, a necessary clinical step, though one that felt painfully redundant at that moment. This is routine. No one expected a different outcome; the absence of a fetal heartbeat had already been established. And yet, the moment was excruciating, a reminder of how even routine procedures can carry a deep emotional toll in the context of loss. The next moments passed by quickly. The couple was told that they could go home and spend some time with their other children before the labour would be induced; however, they decided to stay in the hospital. She was distressed and wanted to give birth as soon as possible.

The medication we gave her to induce labour took effect almost immediately. Since I had been freed from other responsibilities during this shift, I was able to stay with them and offer continuous care. Before her contractions grew strong, we had time to talk. She told me about her pregnancy, how everything had been perfect—no different from her previous pregnancies. She hadn't experienced any stress beyond the usual daily demands and had eaten well and enjoyed being pregnant. At 38 weeks, she had been looking forward to meeting her youngest child soon, the baby who was meant to complete their family, when her routine antenatal visit delivered a shock.

Talking with both of them gave me an opportunity to ask whether they held any beliefs surrounding fetal death. I wanted to understand if they believed in the soul, and if so, how they imagined its progression after death. I've cared for parents who do not believe that a soul continues on, and I speak with them differently than I do with those who hold a belief in an afterlife. In these moments, my task is to honour their worldview, not to assert my own. A single careless comment, no matter how well intentioned, can do lasting harm. They shared with me that they believed their baby would enter paradise after birth, and from there, would watch over and protect them. According to their beliefs, the death of a child in utero is considered profound; they viewed it as an honourable death. This belief, that her baby would dwell in paradise, seemed to shape the mother's presence and her unwavering love throughout labour and birth.

As her contractions became more frequent, there was a stillness in the room, and, in that stillness, I was reminded of one of the things that sets these births apart. Caring for labouring women during a stillbirth is sensorily different than live births. What is always most jarring for me is the absence of any fetal heart monitoring during labour, whether with a handheld doppler or a fetal heart monitor. This means that the vocal toning of the labouring woman during contractions will not be answered by the galloping sounds of fetal heartbeats during the pause between contractions. There is only silence. The birthing room is devoid of auditory fetal presence even before the birth. Even years later, it is a silence I cannot forget.

In the weight of that silence, her labour dynamic became stronger, and I experienced something entirely new. I realised that the birthing body does not pause for heartbreak; it continues its work, even if the baby is no longer alive. I had always imagined that one of the strongest impulses during labour is the physiological connection between the labouring woman and her unborn baby—the mother-baby dyad. On that day, love was the most tangible emotion in the room and existed alongside grief, connecting the mother, the baby, her partner, and me. That feeling of connection, while no longer sustained by the life of the baby, was still strong enough for her to maintain a strong labour dynamic.

After her very last contraction, the quiet in the room was deafening. I did not hold back my tears. Just as I feel joyful and celebrate with parents at the birth of a live baby, I feel the pain and loss for a child who will never know life. The baby looked perfect. We carefully dried her together and then wrapped her in a soft cloth before putting her on her mother's chest. After the birth of the placenta, I quietly left the room while the baby's father recited prayers. The presence of so many emotions in one moment was overwhelming. Can a birth be beautiful and yet not bring forth a new life?

After they had spent some time alone, I returned to the room. They asked if I would bathe their baby with them and wrap her in warm towels afterwards. The presence of the baby seemed to linger in the room throughout the bath and remained as they gently swaddled and then held her, swaying back and forth. The parents stayed for several more hours, holding their child, and saying goodbye in their own time. We parted with a heartfelt embrace. I felt empty and full at the same time. A year later, during a night shift, I answered the bell, and there they were. She was in labour with her rainbow child. This time, our embrace was filled with pure joy. We stood at the door for a moment, taking in the miracle of meeting again.

Dwelling with life and death

Many years after this experience, I was sitting at the breakfast table with my son and my partner. Finally, I was working in a free-standing birth centre, just as I had hoped for when I decided to become a midwife. I had just finished my orientation there and was on-call for the first time as the primary midwife. My 14-year-old asked me bluntly if working at a free-standing birth centre meant that I would not experience stillbirths anymore. I was not sure how to answer that question when my pager went off. I called the client back and heard panic in her voice. She told me that her membranes had ruptured, and her contractions had just started. She was so shaky on the phone that I decided to meet her immediately at the birth centre. We arrived at the same time and went into a birthing room. I first looked for the fetal heartbeats with a handheld doppler, then with the fetal heart monitor. She told me at that point that she had not felt her baby move for days. The ground opened up beneath me, and then beneath them, as we, one after the other, became aware that the baby was no longer alive.

These are moments when midwifery collides with loss. I have had many moments like these when I would have liked to turn back the clock but am called to remain present in the face of irreversible situations, to dwell in a moment that feels excruciating. Heidegger writes of dwelling as a kind of attending, of letting things be as they are, without trying to grasp or control them (1971). He wrote:

Mortals dwell in that they save the earth. ... Saving does not only snatch something from danger. To save really means to set something free in its own presencing. … Mortals dwell in that they receive the sky as sky. They leave to the sun and the moon their journey, to the stars their courses, to the season their blessing and their inclemency; they do not turn night into day nor day into a harassed unrest.

(1971, p. 148)

To *dwell*, in its deepest sense, is not to live in safety or even certainty, but to abide within the fullness of human experience, to pay attention to the world we live in, and, through connection, reveal the profundity of human finitude. Human finitude is not merely the fact that life ends, but the way in which our being is shaped by the awareness that it will, an awareness that grants depth, urgency, and meaning to our encounters, especially in birth and death (Malpas, 2006). For me, to be able to accompany life where it leads, even into sorrow and mystery, has become indelibly an aspect of my identity as a midwife. It did not lead me to a fearful place, but rather to a place where wholeness included a space for emptiness and loss.

A newly qualified midwife's story of stillbirth

During the data collection period of this study, only one newly qualified midwife experienced a stillbirth. When I visited her for her final interview at the birth centre, she asked me not to turn on the digital recorder until she was ready. She wanted to tell me a story but did not know how to begin. Her sorrow filled the room. I understood intuitively that recording a grieving voice is different than recording a joyful one. Stories of grief have their own shape. The timbre of our voice changes. We avoid eye contact. Our words slow down to accommodate the tightening sensation in our throat, as if grief were not permitted to escape from our chest. Sometimes our eyes tear up, both as storyteller and as listener.

There are many ways to approach lived experience in Heideggerian hermeneutic phenomenology. In this case, I turned to poetry, as in Chapter 10. In phenomenological writing, poems render meaning, shaped by the mood in which the experience was told (Green et al., 2021). They can also offer access to the profound emotions that emerge when recounting lived experience, for both the interview partner and the researcher. These emotions often resist the structure of prose. For this reason, I decided not to craft this midwife's experience into a story. The poem, written in the midwife's voice, is shaped as a conversation between her and the woman she cared for, using the midwife's words from her interview.

An Unnecessary Visit

An unnecessary visit
Or so I thought.
Latent phase labour.
I could stay home and sleep,

But you had so many questions,
So, I crawled out of my warm bed to visit you.

In the quiet, cool darkness of a spring night,
Candles burning low in your living room,
I listened to your baby's heart gallop away into the night.
We couldn't know that
Several hours later
It would beat for the last time.

I asked myself afterwards:
When did this happen?
Would she still be here if I had listened longer?
Was there a sign I missed?
What if?
What if?
What if?

She told me:
"You were the last person to listen to her heartbeat."
She said:
"Because of this, I could also listen one more time.
I am grateful that you came."

Now, the weight of her gratitude
Feels like a burden,
Having forever changed
Every heartbeat I will ever hear.

To experience the powerlessness that comes with the realisation that the clock cannot be turned back, and mortality does not wait for the end of a full life, turns each moment of care into an offering. To dwell, in this context, means staying present to what is, not turning away from grief and uncertainty, but also not succumbing to it. It compels us to reconnect to hope and to the enduring belief that presence carries meaning, even in the face of loss.

Becoming in the midst of life and loss

To experience stillbirth is to encounter a fundamental disruption in one's understanding of life. What we come to know in such moments is not alone empirical. The facts surrounding stillbirth, even when they elicit sadness, do not come close to having a lived experience of stillbirth. The affective tone of such moments, the bewilderment, the stillness, and the loss, shape how midwives understand their place in the world and in their work. This chapter has suggested that professional growth in midwifery is much more than the acquisition of theoretical knowledge and technical skills. Profound events compel midwives to open up to new understandings of the profession, understandings that must be owned as such. These moments are often marked by urgency. Stillbirth, though rare, reveals the fragile terrain on which we practice and live.

Therefore, to become a midwife is to dwell with both life and death. It is to carry stories and stillness, to hear not only heartbeats but also be present in their absence, and to move forward with care, including but not expecting all possibilities. The shaping of a midwife's identity cannot be disentangled from these moments. They do not pass through us; we dwell with them.

Questions for reflection

1 How has your understanding of midwifery presence shifted after reading about stillbirth experiences? Consider how presence is expressed when joy is absent and what it means to "dwell" with grief in practice.
2 What emotional responses did this chapter evoke in you, and how might they influence your future approach to loss in midwifery care? Reflect on moments of discomfort, resonance, or awakening.
3 How do you imagine supporting a family through the birth of a stillborn baby while attending to your own emotional well-being?
4 What tools, support systems, or rituals might help you remain present without becoming overwhelmed?
5 In what ways do societal expectations and institutional protocols shape midwives' experiences of stillbirth? How might these structures support or hinder compassionate care?
6 What does it mean for you to "dwell" with both life and death as part of your midwifery identity? Reflect on how carrying stories of both birth and loss may inform your becoming as a midwife.

References

Burden, C., Bradley, S., Storey, C., Ellis, A., Heazell, A. E., Downe, S., Cacciatore, J., & Siassakos, D. (2016, Jan 19). From grief, guilt pain and stigma to hope and pride - A systematic review and meta-analysis of mixed-method research of the psychosocial impact of stillbirth. *BMC Pregnancy Childbirth, 16*, 9. https://doi.org/10.1186/s12884-016-0800-8

Cacciatore, J., & Bushfield, S. (2007). Stillbirth: The mother's experience and implications for improving care. *J Soc Work End Life Palliat Care, 3*(3), 59–79. https://doi.org/10.1300/J457v03n03_06

Green, E., Solomon, M., & Spence, D. (2021). Poem as/and palimpsest: Hermeneutic phenomenology and/as poetic inquiry. *Int J Qual Methods, 20*, 1–9. https://doi.org/10.1177/16094069211053094

Heidegger, M. (1962/2001). *Being and Time* (J. Macquarrie & E. S. Robinson, Trans.; 7th ed.). Blackwell Publishers.

Heidegger, M. (1971). *Poetry, Language, Thought* (1st ed.). Harper & Row.

Kenworthy, D., & Kirkham, M. (2011). *Midwives Coping with Loss and Grief: Stillbirth, Professional and Personal Losses*. Radcliffe Publishing.

Komaromy, C. (2012). Managing emotions at the time of stillbirth and neonatal death. In S. Earle, C. Komaromy, & L. Layne (Eds.), *Understanding Reproductive Loss: Perspectives on Life, Death and Fertility* (pp. 193–203). Ashgate.

Lupton, D. (2012). 'Precious cargo': Foetal subjects, risk and reproductive citizenship. *Crit Public Health, 22*(3), 329–340. https://doi.org/10.1080/09581596.2012.657612

Malpas, J. (2006). *Heidegger's Topology: Being, Place, World*. MIT Press. Table of contents only https://www.loc.gov/catdir/toc/fy0707/2006046709.html

Murphy-Lawless, J. (1998). *Reading Birth and Death: A History of Obstetric Thinking*. Indiana University Press.

Scamell, M. (2011, Nov). The swan effect in midwifery talk and practice: A tension between normality and the language of risk. *Sociol Health Illn, 33*(7), 987–1001. https://doi.org/10.1111/j.1467-9566.2011.01366.x

Thompson, S. (2012). 'As if she never existed': Changing understandings of Perinatal loss in Australia in the twentieth and early twenty-first century. In S. Earle, C. Komaromy, & L. Layne (Eds.), *Understanding Reproductive Loss: Perspectives on Life, Death and Fertility* (pp. 167–178). Ashgate.

12
THE POWER OF REFLECTION
Olivia's story

Introduction

In Chapter 11, we turned towards the profound sorrow of intrauterine death, a form of loss that reshapes the meaning of presence for midwives. Stillbirth bears deep emotional weight in midwifery practice, challenging assumptions about control and certainty. The stories shared illuminated how loss is carried not only by families, but also by midwives, in ways that can alter their sense of responsibility. In learning to dwell with grief, midwives come to a fuller, more human understanding of midwifery care. In this chapter, we follow Olivia, a newly qualified midwife, as she revisits a moment from her training that left her unsettled. Pressured to follow institutional time limits, she felt she did not have time to give due attention to a woman who had disclosed a history of abuse, an action that conflicted with her sense of what midwifery care should be, and, above all, the midwife she wanted to become. During her orientation, she promised herself that she would gift her clients time and compassion.

Kairos and Metanoia: Opportunity, regret, and transformation

The allegory of Kairos and Metanoia offers a frame for Olivia's story, a story shaped by reflection and the ethical weight of missed moments. Kairos, the god of opportunity, has been described as balancing on a wheel or standing on his tiptoes, ready to flee at a moment's notice. His identity is concealed by a long shock of hair that falls across his forehead, while the back of his head is bald, preventing the chance that he could be grabbed once he has passed. He embodies the fleeting nature of opportunities that must be seized when they arrive. Van Manen (2017, p. 821) describes Kairos as "pregnant time," since those charged moments hold potential.

DOI: 10.4324/9781003591306-12

The companion stooped behind Kairos, veiled and silent, is *Metanoia*. As the goddess of remorse and hindsight, she is lesser known in Greek mythology, yet profound in her presence. Metanoia is a compound word composed of *meta* and *nous*, meaning *after* or *beyond* and *mind*. The person who fails to take hold of the Kairos moment comes face to face with Metanoia, who lingers in the shadows of lost opportunity. Where Kairos presents the possibility to be meaningfully present in the moment, Metanoia represents the emotional burden of inaction or inappropriate action that persists after the moment (Myers, 2011). The two form a philosophical pair: one arrives quickly and must be seized without delay; the other lingers afterward, making us aware of regret and shaping how we interpret, remember, and make sense of what has passed. Myers (2011) writes that, in imagery of Metanoia, her gaze is directed within, suggesting more than just repentance. Translated figuratively as afterthought, Metanoia is the embodiment of reflection, offering the chance to look back at what has passed, with the possibility to repent, to amend actions, or to have a change of heart (2011).

Crowther et al. (2015) offer a compelling interpretation of Kairos in the context of childbirth. She describes how moments of birth can pull us beyond structured routines and expected practices, into a space where time is no longer linear and the sacred is felt. In such moments, time is felt and no longer measured. When midwives engage with this dimension of care, they move with the rhythm of Kairos, aware of the subtle, transformative possibilities unfolding in real time. When these moments are missed, the opportunity to connect can be concealed. In midwifery care, this can happen when decisions are rushed without taking time for shared decision-making, or when decisions are based only on guidelines rather than the individual needs of clients. What often remains is the loss of human connection, leading to regret, disappointment, and even sorrow. Carter and Porges (2013, p. 12) write that *disruption in social bonds have ... pervasive consequences for behaviour and physiology.*

This is where Olivia's story begins. Olivia had planned on working in a hospital labour ward after receiving her midwifery certification, but, as her first day of work approached, she began to dread her decision, feeling extreme tension, emotionally and physically. She had a strong impulse to visit a free-standing birth centre before starting to work at the hospital and scheduled a meeting with a midwifery team near her home. She wanted to know what her prospects were and whether she met the criteria to work there. The midwives explained to Olivia that she would be trained and familiarised with midwifery care there over a period of three to four months and would not work alone until she and the team felt she was ready. Olivia's aspirations for midwifery practice included getting to know women during their pregnancy through thorough antenatal care, which she believed should include a psychosocial medical history and ample time to listen to women's concerns and fears. In this sense, the free-standing birth centre fulfilled her ethos of beneficial and benevolent care. Here is Olivia's story of her care of Jane, a woman pregnant with her first child. Olivia's story is crafted out of her three interviews, as well as the voice messages that she sent.

Olivia's story

One of the reasons that I wanted to work at a birth centre was because of an experience that I had at the end of my midwifery studies, you know, when you're not yet finished, but you're more or less allowed to work as if you are finished. Well, I was taking a medical history of a woman at the hospital where my practical training took place. The woman told me something really personal—about having been abused—something that I knew I should discuss with her more deeply, but I couldn't open up space for that. The appointment had to take place within a 15-minute time frame, and I knew that I would be evaluated negatively for not sticking to the appointment schedule. I was only supposed to get basic medical information from her, the kind of information that the hospital thought would be important to know, like: did she have surgery before, does she have allergies, is this her first pregnancy, and so on. In that moment, when I cut her off and moved on to the next subject, I felt that I had cut off a part of her that was really important. What if that part of her story was important to know, to tell, in order for her to have a good birth?

When I started here at the birth centre, it was like being thrown into a totally new world. It's sometimes difficult to take it all in. Knowing what I know now, if I could go back and meet who I was when I started here, I would say: Trust yourself. Express what's inside yourself. I'm grateful every day. I've arrived. I have **always** wanted to do this, even if I didn't know then what **THIS** is. During my midwifery studies, I thought there was something "wrong" with me, not quite right; that the way I see things is wrong; that the way I want to do things is wrong. Maybe the others were right, and I didn't understand what midwives were supposed to do. But then I started working at the birth centre, and I felt so free.

I've experienced so many good births, easy births here, but one of the births that was the most amazing was Jane's birth, a woman who didn't actually give birth here. I ended up having to transfer her to the hospital, and it changed how I saw the birth centre. My care for her started in a morning shift. Jane had already been at the birth centre the whole night. The birth was moving along slowly. When she had contractions, I was in awe of her strength. What was really exceptional about her was that she fought so hard to let go. That's what I felt.

This is what happened: She had this rhythm during labour where she would shut down, then she would throw up and, after that, she would let go and blossom, and the birth would move forward. Then she would shut down again. This happened every two hours. I asked what might help her, and she said that she liked to sing and dance at home. So, she asked her husband to put on the song Let it Go from Frozen. I left the birthing room, and they sang and danced together. After a while, I came back into the room, and we danced around the room together.

I was in awe of her courage, but also frustrated and sad. I eventually had to transfer her. She was exhausted and the baby wasn't descending into the birth canal. She was totally relieved when she was transferred and asked for a cesarean section at the hospital, even though the doctor at the hospital was certain that she could give birth easily with an epidural (pain relief) and an oxytocin drip (augmentation of the contractions). But Jane felt she had worked hard and tried everything and was ready to have her baby. I can't even explain how frustrated I felt after this, but I visited her at home (a month) after the birth and had an intense talk with her.

I thought she would be sad, but she told me that she was a different person than she was before the birth. She can express herself now. She can tell people what she is feeling. She was never able to do this before her birth. I was so astonished. Her labour here at the birth centre—it was good for that. She didn't have to actually give birth here. In a way, she gave birth to herself and has come out of her shell. And she was happy with the cesarean section, and that she had made the decision herself.

That's why there are birth centres. It's not about how many women actually give birth here. It's about giving women a space to go their own way. Even if we can only accompany a woman part of the way, and then she gets to the moment where she can't go on here, then that's okay. If she needed the care from us for part of her labour and then decides to give birth in the hospital, then that's what we're here for. If she feels good here, then she should be here. We're not here to tally births. We can't and don't look at everything through rose-coloured glasses. I don't anymore.

Standing in Metanoia's shadow: Becoming through reflection

Metanoia, associated with regret, can also signal the emergence of a new way of thinking, as it did for Olivia. Her postnatal conversation with Jane became a turning point, guiding her towards a deeper understanding of her role as a midwife. She no longer measured the value or virtue of her care by the location or mode of birth. What gained significance instead were the connections formed during antenatal appointments; the moments during labour where relational presence makes a difference; and the lasting experience of birth in the lives of each woman and baby. While she still saw value in vaginal birth where possible, she let go of the notion that it was the sole hallmark of a good birth. In the process of letting go, she began to see care differently and moved closer to being able to practice midwifery in a way that aligned with her beliefs.

Releasing old conceptions and approaches often requires profound reflection and takes courage. During her interview, Olivia asked me to put on the song "Let it go" (Lopez & Anderson-Lopez, 2013) from the movie *Frozen*, the music that Jane danced to with her husband during labour. Hearing it for the first time, I was struck by how the lyrics captured both women's inner landscapes and resonated with the performative expectations that many student midwives carry into practice from institutional training, such as being a good girl, as well as the performative expectations of labouring women (Martin, 2003). For Olivia, letting go of preconceived, unattainable ambitions was not achieved in a Kairos moment. To transform, she needed Metanoia.

While conducting research over the years in free-standing birth centres, I have often heard midwives tell stories in which the theme of redemption surfaces. These stories often follow a familiar pattern: as a student or newly qualified midwife in a hospital, she witnessed or took part in care that she felt caused harm. Unable to undo the damage or make amends to the woman affected, she made a promise to herself to never again be part of such disrespect. That promise becomes a kind of living reparation, carried forward in her care for others. The power of Metanoia, as reflection and afterthought, is the possibility she brings to humans to co-create and build a better world.

Olivia felt that she was the best midwife she could be in her care of Jane, yet it seemed, at first, to be a failed attempt. When the birth is experienced as the end of the story, and a vaginal birth at the birth centre is envisaged as the crowning moment, then transfer to the hospital seems like a bitter pill to swallow. Olivia doubted herself and the birth centre for a brief period of time, as well as her ability to make good on the harm she witnessed and caused in her clinical placement during her studies. Yet in revisiting the experience with Jane, Olivia recognised that the moment of transfer had not undermined her care but had revealed the complexity of what it means to be a midwife committed to relational practice in a free-standing birth centre, where transfer of clients is a necessity for some women.

Meeting clinical expectations

Midwifery students are expected to fulfil specified criteria in the clinical settings where they train. As with any form of practical learning, expectations can conflict with lived experience. In the gap between what one hopes to do and what one is required to do, when rule-following overrides the impulse to connect in order to be a good student, seeds of self-doubt or even shame may be sown. This happened with Olivia when she was not allowed to break the 15-minute rule for appointments. When she moved on too quickly after a woman disclosed a history of abuse, she felt she had cut off something vital, something that might have mattered for the woman's upcoming birth. For Olivia, that moment had staying power. Skimming past what mattered felt like a betrayal, not just of the woman, but of her own sense of what good, ethical midwifery care should be. In that moment, she felt that she had cut off part of the woman. Listening to Olivia tell this story, I had the sense that she had also cut off part of herself. When she began her orientation, her feeling of inner repose returned that lost part. Reflecting on what might have helped her during her training, Olivia imagined her current self going back in time to say: "Trust yourself. Keep going. You'll get there." This, too, is the essence of Metanoia, when a shift in perception and subsequent actions takes place.

Embodied reflection and relational becoming

While Heidegger (1926/2006) does not foreground the body in the same way Merleau-Ponty (1958) later would, his explorations in *Being and Time* imply a form of *being-in-the-world* as embodied existence. Dasein is not a detached mind observing the world, but a being-in-the-world whose orientation is always already shaped by thrownness, attunement, and care. These structures (in German *Geworfenheit*, *Befindlichkeit*, and *Sorge*) are fundamentally corporeal (physical), even if Heidegger refrains from detailing how the body figures in these structures. Polt (1999, p. 57) writes:

> [Existence] occurs when the human body interacts with the beings around it in such a way that those beings reveal themselves in their depths of meaning. If our connections to other beings were cut, we would not end up inside our mind – we would end up without a mind at all.

By contrast, Merleau-Ponty places embodiment at the core of his phenomenology, arguing that the lived body (*le corps propre*) is not a thing among things but that by which the world becomes available to perception. Merleau-Ponty (1957, p. 146) writes: *The body is our general medium for having a world.* This means that the body is the site where perception and meaning are always already intertwined. As such, meaning shows up *with* our bodily experience. Taken together, these perspectives articulate how midwifery care unfolds through co-responsive bodily presence and intentional care, in addition to learned, abstract, theoretical constructs. Through the body's capacity to see, touch, hear, and move, we are always engaged with the world in a meaningful way. Merleau-Ponty describes this as lived perception, a bodily awareness that is not directed towards meaning as something separate but is already immersed in the meaningfulness of the world.

This explanation helps clarify why it takes time for newly qualified midwives to orient themselves towards offering embodied forms of care. They learn to broaden their clinical judgement, which, at the end of their studies, was largely based on measurable data. Over time, this judgement comes to include lived perception: how the woman speaks, moves, breathes, and responds to her environment and the people in it. It also involves how the midwife, in turn, listens, touches, observes, and even smells within that shared space. These sensory and affective dimensions are not subordinate to clinical facts, and clinical measures are absolutely not omitted in care in free-standing birth centres; rather, they operate in concert with them, each informing the other. Reflection then allows midwives to become aware of the meaning already present in these encounters and to respond with care that is both clinical and attuned to lived experience. This interplay between perception and reflection also opens a way to understand how moments of care can carry an ethical weight that is *felt* before it is articulated, and regretted, when it is missed.

Moral emotions and the biology of becoming

Insights from social psychology and neuroscience offer a way to understand Olivia's experience and others like it as examples of how moral emotions arise. Human beings experience emotions in response to events that involve them personally, even if they are just witnesses. According to Haidt (2003, p. 854), emotions triggered by social interactions, especially during triumphs, tragedies, and transgressions, are typically moral in nature. These moral emotions arise in response to observing acts of suffering, injustice, kindness, or beauty, and often evoke, e.g., anger, guilt, compassion, or elevation. Moral emotion moves people to care for, uphold, or strengthen the world they live in, even when the actions it inspires are not necessarily kind, as in the case of revenge-seeking. Haidt organises these emotions into what he calls "emotion families," each defined by a core set of emotions, particular eliciting conditions, and their associated action tendencies. (See Table 12.1).

Further, moral emotions function as "commitment devices," whereby people tend to commit to action that will support well-being in the longer term (Haidt, 2003, p. 854). One such emotion is moral elevation, a concept introduced by Haidt

TABLE 12.1 Haidt's Moral Emotion Families

Emotion Family	Core Emotions	Eliciting Conditions	Action Tendencies/ Functions
Other-condemning	Contempt, anger, disgust (plus indignation, loathing)	Perception of moral violations, unfairness, betrayal, degradation	Punish, distance, condemn, restore social/moral order
Self-conscious	Shame, embarrassment, guilt	Awareness of having violated norms or harmed others	Withdrawal, self-correction, repair, appeasement
Other-suffering	Compassion	Perception of others in distress or suffering	Help, comfort, relieve suffering
Other-praising	Gratitude, elevation	Witnessing moral beauty or virtue in others	Approach, emulate virtue, strengthen social bonds, inspire moral growth

Adapted from Haidt (2003, p. 855)

(2000) to describe the feeling people experience when they witness acts of human goodness, compassion, or virtue. Importantly, the internal resources developed during episodes of positive emotion have enduring effects and outlast the fleeting emotional states that gave rise to them (Fredrickson & Branigan, 2005). These resources can serve as reserves, available for future use to facilitate coping, adaptation, and resilience. An explanation for this might be that positive emotions of joy and strength, felt during acts of kindness, orient us towards doing more of the same, informing and guiding our intentions in the future.

Understanding how such emotions leave a physiological and motivational imprint brings us to the question of what happens in the body during these moments. To explore this further, recent findings from social neuroscience offer valuable insights, suggesting that emotions are also fundamentally neurobiological events, as evidenced in the foundational work by Carter on the neuroendocrine role of oxytocin (Carter, 1998; Carter & Porges, 2013; Carter et al., 2020). Carter has shown that oxytocin plays a central role in supporting social bonding, emotional regulation, and physiological calm, what she and colleagues (2020) have described as "nature's medicine." Olivia's story exemplifies how such a transformation may occur through embodied, emotionally significant experiences that have an effect on physiology.

Research by Zak (2015), who refers to oxytocin as the "moral molecule," demonstrates that emotionally meaningful narratives can stimulate oxytocin release, enhancing empathy, trust, and, prosocial behaviour. While his studies often involve exposing research participants to emotionally charged scenes in films, his findings point to underlying neurochemical mechanisms that are equally relevant in real-life, lived experiences. Hammond et al. (2014), whose research centres on birth environments, also propose that oxytocin plays a key role in fostering trust and connection. In other words, emotionally attuned caregiving moments and reflective professional encounters may activate similar neurochemical pathways. Together, these findings suggest that Olivia's transformation was a plausible outcome of offering relational care, in which positive moral emotions and embodied connection resulted in neurophysiological safety.

Meaningful care

Olivia's experience invites us to consider how midwifery is shaped when expectations feel unethical. Her story reveals the weight of moments that slip past; in particular how institutional demands can close down opportunities for connection, and how such closures linger in memory, influencing the kind of midwife one longs to become. In a setting that encouraged reflection, Olivia discovered that care is best when time is made for engagement. What matters in these moments is presence: the capacity to remain with what is unfolding, even when it leads away from the imagined path. In practice, this means recognising that good midwifery cannot be measured by economic efficiency or mode of birth. It lives in the complexity of relationship, in embodied encounters, and in the reflective work that follows, where the meaning of care continues to take shape.

Questions for reflection

1 How do institutional structures shape what is possible—or impossible—in moments of care, and how might midwives navigate these tensions without losing their ethical grounding?
2 What does Olivia's story reveal about the role of reflection in transforming past regret into future orientation?
3 How can midwives cultivate the capacity to stay present in situations that do not resolve neatly or follow expected paths?
4 In what ways does relational presence, rather than outcome, serve as a meaningful measure of good midwifery care? Is there a part of you that you feel is cut off when you cannot give the care that you think should be given?
5 How might missed moments, when approached reflectively, become formative rather than merely wounding in a midwife's development?

References

Carter, S. C. (1998). Neuroendicrine perspectives on social attachment and love. *PNE, 23*(8), 779–818. https://doi.org/10.1016/s0306-4530(98)00055-9

Carter, S. C., Kenkel, W. M., MacLean, E. L., Wilson, S. R., Perkeybile, A. M., Yee, J. R., Ferris, C. F., Nazarloo, H. P., Porges, S. W., Davis, J. M., Connelly, J. J., & Kingsbury, M. A. (2020). Is oxytocin "nature's medicine"? *Pharmacol Rev, 72*, 829–861. https://doi.org/10.1124/pr.120.019398

Carter, S. C., & Porges, S. W. (2013). The biochemistry of love: An oxytocin hypothesis: Science & society series on sex and science. *EMBO Rep, 14*, 12–16. https://doi.org/10.1038/embor.2012.191

Crowther, S., Smythe, E., & Spence, D. (2015, Apr). Kairos time at the moment of birth. *Midwifery, 31*(4), 451–457. https://doi.org/10.1016/j.midw.2014.11.005

Fredrickson, B. L., & Branigan, C. (2005, May 1). Positive emotions broaden the scope of attention and thought-action repertoires. *Cogn Emot, 19*(3), 313–332. https://doi.org/10.1080/02699930441000238

Haidt, J. (2000). The positive emotion of elevation. *Prev Treat, 3*, 1–5. https://doi.org/10.1037/1522-3736.3.1.33c

Haidt, J. (2003). The moral emotions. In R. J. Davidson, K. R. Scherer, & H. H. Goldsmith (Eds.), *Handbook of Affective Sciences* (pp. 852–870). Oxford University Press.

Hammond, A. D., Homer, C. E., & Foureur, M. (2014, Summer). Messages from space: An exploration of the relationship between hospital birth environments and midwifery practice. *HERD, 7*(4), 81–95. https://doi.org/10.1177/193758671400700407

Heidegger, M. (1926/2006). *Sein und Zeit*. Max Niemeyer Verlag.

Lopez, R., & Anderson-Lopez, K. (2013). Let it go [Song]. On *Frozen Soundtrack [Film]*. Walt Disney Records.

Martin, K. A. (2003). Giving birth like a girl. *Gender & Society, 17*(1), 54–72. https://www.jstor.org/stable/3081814

Merleau-Ponty, M. (1958). *Phenomenology of Perception* (C. Smith, Trans.). Routledge Classics.

Myers, K. A. (2011). Metanoia and the transformation of opportunity. *RSQ, 41*(1), 1–18. https://doi.org/10.1080/02773945.2010.533146

Polt, R. (1999). *Heidegger: An Introduction* (Kindle ed.). Routledge.

van Manen, M. (2017, May). Phenomenology in its original sense. *Qual Health Res, 27*(6), 810–825. https://doi.org/10.1177/1049732317699381

Zak, P. J. (2015, Jan-Feb). Why inspiring stories make us react: The neuroscience of narrative. *Cerebrum, 2015*, 2. https://www.ncbi.nlm.nih.gov/pubmed/26034526

13

"I AM THE MIDWIFE I DREAMED OF BECOMING"

Amelia's story

In Chapter 12, we followed Olivia as she reflected on an unsettling encounter during her clinical training. That moment was formative, influencing her choice to work in a free-standing birth centre and offer relational care. Her story illustrated how regret, when reflected upon and acted on, can transform work ethic and emotional presence. Through the lens of Kairos and Metanoia, it became clear how missed or unsettling moments can be an impetus for professional growth. In this chapter, we follow Amelia across her three interviews conducted during her first year in a free-standing birth centre, each marking a different stage in her orientation as a newly qualified midwife. Her story unfolds in her own words, revealing her development of clinical skill across that first year. The Dreyfus model of skill acquisition and Porges' Polyvagal Theory provide a framework for understanding how her growth was supported by relational care and clinical presence. These theories offer background context; however, this chapter is driven primarily by Amelia's narrative.

A place to begin: Professional becoming in a safe environment

Hubert Dreyfus and Stuart Dreyfus' (1980) model of skill acquisition outlines a five-stage progression from novice to expert (novice, competence, proficiency, expertise, mastery) specifically developed to describe skill acquisition of pilots. This framework has since been widely applied to other fields, most notably in nursing, where Patricia Benner (1984) adapted the Dreyfus framework to describe the experiential learning process of nurses. Drawing on an updated version of the model (Dreyfus, 1981), she renamed stages as: novice, advanced beginner, competent, proficient, and expert. Dreyfus and Dreyfus (1980) challenged the assumption that expertise arises solely from rational

DOI: 10.4324/9781003591306-13

analysis or rule-based decision-making. Instead, they emphasised the gradual integration of tacit knowledge, embodied responsiveness, and context-sensitive understanding (Dreyfus & Dreyfus, 2005). Hubert Dreyfus later referred to this process as "skilful coping" (2014). While the model does not fully capture the relational, embodied, and contextually nuanced nature of skill acquisition in midwifery practice, it provides a useful heuristic (interpretive) framework to reference the established trajectory of skill development, supporting reflection on the experiential transitions that shape the newly qualified midwives' paths through orientation. In addition to this, applying the model, albeit loosely, reveals the distinctive nature of midwifery practice.

In the novice stage, learners are introduced to what the Dreyfus model (1980, p. 7) calls a "decomposed task environment," in which foundational tasks are abstracted from the broader situation and presented as non-situational elements, basic components that must be learned in order to grasp the general aim of the activity. Examples of non-situational elements in midwifery are, e.g., introducing oneself to a client, performing hand hygiene (including maintaining short fingernails), tying back one's hair, asking permission before touching, and following procedural checklists. Actions such as these are tied to explicit rules, and performance is dependent on following these rules correctly. At the start of her orientation, Amelia was situated within the novice stage in the context of the free-standing birth centre, as the setting was new to her; however, she already demonstrated attributes of the advanced beginner stage, attributes that she had developed through clinical placements undertaken during her education.

The early weeks of observation at the birth centre were designed to help Amelia become familiar with the rules and routines of the setting. This included, for example, learning how to conduct antenatal examinations according to gestational age, a task that varied depending on the week of pregnancy. In the advanced beginner stage, the learner is placed in real-life situations and learns to cope with the demands of the work environment, relying on guidelines to facilitate decision-making. As Dreyfus and Dreyfus (1980) note, it is through repeated engagement in a particular context that the learner's perception begins to shift, marking the gradual move beyond rule-dependence. This can only be attained in real-life situations.

When viewed through this lens, Amelia's first interview reveals a clear movement along this continuum. Her arc of lived experience also reveals a shift from fear, nervousness, and emotional uncertainty towards a sense of physiological and embodied safety. Polyvagal Theory (Porges, 2011) helps us understand how the ethos of the free-standing birth centre and the support of her mentors and colleagues functioned as a regulatory environment; a place where her nervous system, no longer in defensive overdrive as it was so often in her clinical training, could support skill acquisition and a growing love for her profession. The table below, adapted from Porges (2011, 2022), presents key terms and definitions that inform the interpretation of Amelia's lived experience (Table 13.1).

TABLE 13.1 Understanding the Nervous System's Role in Learning and Becoming

Term	Definition	How It Appears in Amelia's Story
Neuroception	The nervous system's unconscious ability to detect safety, danger, or life threat.	Amelia's nervous system initially senses the hospital as threatening, even without overt danger. In contrast, the birth centre feels safe before she can explain why.
Ventral vagal state	A state of physiological calm and social engagement; supports learning, connection, and presence.	This state gradually emerges in Amelia's story as she begins to feel accepted, supported, and capable of relational midwifery care.
Sympathetic activation	A state of mobilisation associated with fight or flight responses to perceived threat.	Amelia's rushed reactions, fear of being judged, and anxiety during early hospital experiences, as well as during transfers, reflect sympathetic overdrive.
Dorsal vagal state	A shutdown state marked by disconnection, helplessness, numbness, or collapse.	During her clinical training and in one situation at the birth centre, Amelia describes a painful withdrawal and the inability to ask questions or interject her opinion, a classic dorsal state.
Co-regulation	The process through which the nervous system downregulates defensive states via consistent, supportive social interaction.	Amelia's colleagues offer steady relational cues that foster safety, helping her nervous system shift from defence to engagement and learning. Over time, Amelia herself begins to co-regulate clients by modulating her presence to support their sense of safety during care interactions.
Safe environment	A context in which neuroception facilitates the detection of cues of safety, allowing the autonomic nervous system to down-regulate defence responses and support social engagement, reflection, and growth.	For Amelia, the birth centre becomes a safe environment: a setting that promotes physiological calm and supports her development as a midwife.

Adapted from Stephen Porges (2011, 2022)

The first interview

In Amelia's first interview, the distress left over from her hospital training is still active. She recalls how, in her clinical training, the relational environment felt so toxic to her that it hindered her ability to learn. Her clinical midwifery practice as a student was shaped to a greater extent by anxiety rather than engagement. What follows is her lived experience of the first six weeks of her orientation, including how she began to make sense of her prior experiences as she began her orientation in her free-standing birth centre.

Amelia's first six weeks

The last year of my training was awful because of the issues that I had at the hospital where I did my clinical training. I felt terrible most of the time and never wanted to see a pregnant person ever again. Never. It was physically painful—it went that deep. I felt like I was the annoying student tagging along—someone they had to deal with but preferred not to. There was zero tolerance for not knowing something instantly. At the beginning of my fifth semester, I just couldn't handle it anymore. I had an experience during a shift where I needed a moment to think—just a moment—and, instead of someone saying to me: "It's okay. Ask me what you want to know," she insulted me. Eventually, I didn't dare ask any questions anymore. Sometimes I would secretly go into an empty room, take out my phone, and google things because I was too afraid to ask anyone.

I thought that the atmosphere might be different in a birth centre. I still remember when I came here for a visit to spend a day observing the midwives and to interview with them. I arrived thinking, "Okay, behave yourself, be quiet. It's best if you don't say anything" and then Katharina, one of the midwives, came up to me and said, "Hey, Amelia, it's so nice to meet you! How are you? Tell me about yourself." And I was just like—wow. These people are actually engaging with me, and I found out that one of the goals here is to get to know each other and to build strong, trusting relationships.

So, I got the job here, and, in the first weeks I noticed that I really enjoyed being a midwife. The learning environment here is safe. My mentor said to me when I started: "You're going to make a lot of mistakes; maybe the same one more than once. And eventually, you won't anymore. Just keep asking us until you get it." That's a really good feeling. If I make a mistake here—forget to check a box or don't know where something is, no one throws it in my face. They don't insult me. And, even more than that, when I leave the birth centre to go home, I am in awe of how many beautiful interactions I've had with people. What blows me away the most is the atmosphere at births. [I've been here for 6 weeks now and] I haven't seen the whole process of what the midwife does to create that incredible atmosphere, but I think it's partly the space—the birthing rooms here are lovely—but also the mood, maybe her mood? Maybe it's just the birth itself? I don't know yet.

When I get a call to come to the birth centre, my initial feeling is stress—adrenaline. I have to rush around and pack my things, jump on my bicycle and pedal to the birth centre. I arrive totally sweaty, change my clothes, and put on my work shoes. And then I have to do a 180° turn emotionally—I have to let go of all the stress and tension that I brought with me before I can even think about entering the birthing room. I have to align myself with the "birth mood," which is calm and somehow protective, like a cocoon. It's like a place between worlds or another world. And I can totally feel that even before I enter the room. I already feel it the moment I'm standing in front of the door and thinking: Now I'm entering another world. It's a lovely feeling, when I softly knock on the door, press down the door handle, tiptoe in, check to see if anyone looks up at me, and give a little wave. Sometimes I say, "Hi, I'm Amelia, the second midwife," or the first midwife will introduce me and say: "This is Amelia, the second midwife. I already told you about her." I smile at the people in the room and then quietly walk to my place, sit down, and, if my colleague doesn't need anything from me, I just observe.

Before births, when I'm riding to the birth centre on my bicycle or taking public transportation, I wish I could just scream it to the world: "Do you all know where I'm going? I have the most amazing job. I'm a midwife and am on my way to the birth centre for a birth!" After births, when I'm on my way home, the urge is even stronger. I want to tell everyone: "Do you know where I just was? I was at a birth in the birth centre." I want everyone to know the miracle I witnessed. That I'm not coming from the office or the university or whatever—I AM A MIDWIFE.

I wish I could say that every moment has been great, but that's not the case. Early on in my orientation, I was at a birth where we had to transfer a woman during labour to the hospital. My colleague wanted me to go with, since I hadn't seen a transfer yet. I felt kind of sick to my stomach and must have sighed really loud because my colleague asked me if I had a "hospital trauma." I was so relieved that she said it out loud. I looked at her and said: YES—and then I was okay—as if I only needed to say it out loud. My colleague didn't take my experience for granted. She knew how I felt and that reassured me. The best part was that, when we got to the hospital, everyone there was so nice. My colleague introduced me and said I was in my orientation. The midwife at the hospital took note of my name and spoke to me directly. It was a really good experience.

One thing I keep coming back to is this transition—this question of, what kind of midwife am I going to be? Until now, it's only been about what kind of student midwife I was. And now I have to figure it out. That seems to be a part of orientation, this switch from being a student midwife to being a full-on midwife. That's what's happening.

Amelia spoke a great deal about the atmosphere during births in the birthing room in all of her interviews, something that seemed vital for the development of sensory-based skills for all of the newly qualified midwives in this study. Amelia's reflections also draw attention to the powerful role of atmosphere in shaping early professional identity. While Dreyfus and Dreyfus and Benner focus on context-appropriate, situated action, Polyvagal Theory (Porges, 2011) highlights how relational cues of safety foster the physiological conditions necessary for presence and connection. Although Porges does not frame his work in terms of learning, his emphasis on safety and co-regulation offers a useful lens for understanding how supportive environments might enable the kind of reflective practice Amelia begins to describe in her next interview.

The second interview

By the time of the second interview, Amelia had progressed to working as the second midwife without an experienced midwife as backup. She felt less threatened in her day-to-day role at the birth centre, suggesting that ongoing co-regulation was contributing to the reduction of her instances of sympathetic activation (Porges, 2011). Unlike during her midwifery studies, she no longer described slipping into a dorsal vagal state, which is marked by shutdown and helplessness (Porges, 2011). As her tasks at the birth centre became more familiar, her anxiety decreased in most situations. No longer operating under threat, she was able to perceive cues of trust and support.

When we met, she was on-call as first midwife for her first client. Her lived experience six months into her orientation revealed a shift from advanced beginner towards competent practitioner, as described in Benner's model of skill acquisition (1984). While, according to Benner, full competence typically develops after two to three years of clinical experience, Amelia's stories demonstrate an accelerated development likely shaped by the emotionally safe and supportive environment of the birth centre; the model of care in which she cares for only one labouring woman at a time; and her nourishing relationships with her colleagues. Her descriptions reflect deliberate, responsible action, embodied decision-making, and an emerging clinical intuition, all characteristics of the competent stage.

Amelia's first six months

Hmm, what's changed? I've become more self-confident and am much more comfortable now at antenatal appointments with clients. The conversation flows better. I don't have to stick so rigidly to a script anymore because now I know that if I lose the thread, I can find my way back. And in the end, I know—okay, I've said everything I needed to say. I know what clients have to know and have time to go off on tangents if that's where they want to go. So that makes me more relaxed. And I've been second midwife for months now and am not nervous about it at all anymore because, well, it's birth—and that's incredible—but somehow,

I have the feeling that, as second midwife, I feel really comfortable. I'm not on shaky ground anymore. I'm on solid footing and ready to be first midwife.

I had a huge realisation not too long ago. At a birth where I was second midwife, I noticed that I still expect my colleague to take on most of the responsibility, and I suddenly understood that that has to change. For sure, I trust the midwives to make sound clinical judgements, make the right decisions, and carry the responsibility. It's not about that. I still saw myself as someone who just came to assist the first midwife, but not anymore. I am just as responsible for our client and the baby as the first midwife, especially in an emergency. Since then, I've been so, uhm—it's hard to explain. I was at a home birth and, as the second midwife, I do things like get the warm towels when the baby is born. We had a client who wanted to be alone with the baby after she gave birth and not have people around her making noise. So, I simply laid the towel on the baby without helping her dry it, but I noticed that that left me feeling uncertain because, usually, when I dry the baby, I notice the baby's muscle tone and reflexes. I felt like I had missed something by not getting that tactile impression. I knew that my first midwife had gone through the whole Apgar scheme – she was the one who caught the baby and saw that it was breathing normally and was fit and rosy. At first, I wasn't really sure if I could just let go of it and accept that my colleague was checking that the baby was adapting well. After a few minutes, I was so uncomfortable that I finally went ahead and told our client that I needed to check the baby. I was missing that sensation of checking the baby's muscle tone. It's one of the ways that I know that the baby is "here." I hadn't even really seen the baby yet; and I hadn't felt how it responds to my touch. So, I grabbed another warm towel and laid it on the baby. In that moment, I put both hands lightly on the baby and felt it respond. And then I felt calm. That was a great moment, to realise: if something is missing for me to get the whole picture of how mom and baby are doing, I have to check it out. I need to make sure that I feel good in the situation, too, and not just rely on my colleague.

I was also at an incredibly moving birth recently. I was resting at home after having been at a birth during the night. In the afternoon, I got a call to come to the birth centre. When I got there, our client was in the birthing pool. She was really pushing intensely. She wasn't just bearing down a little—she was vocalising at full volume with her whole face clenched, biting her teeth together—her face was bright red. She was really pressing—not just pushing lightly, she was pressing with everything she had. Sitting in the tub with her legs bent, it seemed as if, even between contractions, she was still feeling the remnants of the contraction before. She was just totally consumed with it all.

As second midwife, I wasn't actively doing anything. I just sat quietly and did the documentation, observing these two very strikingly beautiful people who were about to become parents. Yeah, just a really beautiful couple. So, the scene itself—this incredibly beautiful woman with a contorted face pushing her baby out—it was a breath-taking moment. And then the baby was born. The woman reached into the water and lifted the baby out herself and immediately started crying. From emotion. She started sobbing right away, saying things like, "You're so beautiful," and immediately speaking to the baby. We all ended up crying. I cried, my colleague cried, and her partner—he cried too. We were all just in awe. It was this contrast between the intense effort and pain she had just been through and this instant shift into deep emotion and enchantment—it was just too much, in the best way. We all shed tears and really treasured the moment.

Amelia's lived experience of births in her second interview shows a departure from Dreyfus' and Benner's models. While Benner's (1984) model outlines a gradual movement towards competence over years of clinical exposure, it is important to consider the contextual differences between hospital-based nursing and midwifery care in free-standing birth centres. Midwives working in settings like Amelia's attend to one client at a time, allowing for focused, relational, and often uninterrupted care. This continuity enables the midwife to maintain a view of the whole, as her attention is not repeatedly diverted by competing demands. Within this environment, Amelia demonstrates embodied responsiveness and emerging intuitive judgement that more closely resemble elements of proficient practice than what would typically be expected at this stage. Her growing ability to interpret complex clinical moments and act confidently suggests that context and continuity of care can accelerate the development of situated expertise.

The third interview

In her third interview, Amelia had been first midwife for almost six months. She now bears full clinical responsibility in moments that are both routine and urgent, working independently on a regular basis. No longer a novice needing explicit instruction, she is increasingly able to respond quickly and remain calm. In this last interview, she reflected on judgement, timing, and the tension she felt when having to hand over a complex situation to a more experienced colleague, a moment where she once again fell into a dorsal vagal state of shutdown. She also shares her uplifting experience when she suddenly became aware that she was the midwife she had dreamed of becoming.

Amelia's first year

I've been first midwife for around 6 months now. I really want to tell you about the transfers. I had so many. They're super emotional for me but on a different level. So, my first transfer as first midwife was the first time I transferred a client to a hospital without another colleague with me. I had been at the birth centre with this client already for almost twelve hours earlier that week. Then, the contractions stopped; the baby was doing fine; and the cervix was about three to four centimetres dilated. We decided that she should go home. Two days later, she got contractions again and came back to the birth centre. We spent another twelve hours at the birth centre—until, again the contractions went away. We decided together it was time to transfer to the hospital because she was simply exhausted. She ended up having a c-section hours later. Honestly, on the one hand, it was awful for me, because going to the hospital without the protection of another colleague made me anxious. But, on the other hand, when it was over, it felt kind of empowering because I survived it. I thought, okay—I managed everything, and mom and baby were good. I got through it, and they actually took me seriously there.

A few days after that, I had another transfer. This time, it was during the active phase of labour, and we had late decelerations down to 60 bpm, so I called the EMTs, and we had an urgent transfer by ambulance. I wasn't alone at the birth centre and had help organising everything, making all the phone calls, and getting our client ready. It was my first time riding in an ambulance.

Then there was the third transfer, which has really stuck with me. When this client first called during the day, I decided to visit her at home. At that point, she didn't have regular contractions, so she stayed home. Later that evening, when her contractions were regular, she and her partner came to the birth centre. Her labour progressed pretty steadily. She was in the water and really working hard. Eventually, when she went into transition, I called my second midwife. When my colleague arrived, our client already had an incredibly intense urge to push—like her whole body was bearing down. At one point we could see the head between the labia, but it never got beyond that point. We kept changing positions over and over. At some point, I felt overwhelmed. My second midwife and I didn't discuss out loud that we would change roles. I simply glanced at her helplessly, and she understood that she should take over. I didn't take back the lead after that.

She took a more direct approach than I had and did a perineal massage, somehow trying to manoeuvre the baby down at the same time. My colleague checked in with our client just as each contraction started and asked for her permission to do this massage and she was okay with it. And, even though I wasn't the one doing the perineal massage, and even though our client said it was okay, I was still there, and it made me really uncomfortable to witness it. It felt like the baby was coming any second, but it just wasn't working. At some point, we all agreed that it was time to transfer. We transferred with an ambulance, and the baby was born via vacuum extraction. She had thick meconium-stained amniotic fluid, and the baby had the cord looped around her neck with her hand inside the loop! The heartbeats had been fine all along—the baby hadn't shown any signs of distress. I had even done a CTG. We wouldn't have stayed at the birth centre if that hadn't been the case.

I had to really reflect on what had bothered me so much. Was it that I had given up the lead? Was it the perineal massage, which seemed really intense to me? Even though it wasn't me doing it at that point, I was still there, and I shared responsibility for the whole situation. It almost felt like some of the difficult births I witnessed during my [hospital] training, where I felt like I was on the wrong side of it all. I don't know what to think at this point except that I don't see myself doing a perineal massage like that any time soon.

After that, I was thinking—I've had so many transfers—shit. There's no point in trying to give birth with me because I'll just end up transferring you. Better not do it. Of course, I never said that out loud, but I did start thinking it. And then I actually had ANOTHER transfer. I was with a labouring client in the birth centre—and, for hours, everything was going well. In all of my transfers up until that one, I wasn't alone in the birth centre. Either I had enough time to call my second midwife, and we made the decision together, or it was during the day, and there were plenty of colleagues in the birth centre to help me. But at this birth, during a routine check of the fetal heartbeats, they dropped to 90 bpm, and I was alone. Even after moving my client into a different position, they were still at 90 bpm. I checked her pulse, which was higher. I had a deep sense of what it means to be alone at that moment and thought—you can do this. I told my client that I needed to transfer her and called for an ambulance. And then I did everything after that like clockwork. I called emergency services— listened to the fetal heartbeats again—which were now normal—called the labour ward at the transfer hospital and called my second midwife. While I was dialling the phone, I told my client to get her insurance ID and pregnancy record book ready and asked her partner to help her get dressed. I didn't even have to think about the steps—they were a part of me. It was a tense situation, but I already felt better because the baby had recovered. That was a relief. I rode in the ambulance, and I could do report—give all the details—without pause. My senses were heightened the whole time. And I actually had a really good experience talking to the emergency physician who was riding with us. I just knew exactly what needed to be done, and that felt amazing to know deeply: I can do this now. And I had had so many transfers at that point that everyone at the hospital said: "Wait—we've seen you here a few times already." And I said, "Yup, I'm kind of on a roll right now. Hopefully we won't see each other again for a while." And then they said, "Yeah, but you do good transfers. You bring us the right cases at the right time."

I was really confident after that. All those non-urgent transfers before the most recent one had prepared me to know exactly what to do in an emergency. How amazing is that? And something I've learned through all this—especially during the last two births—that I also need to feel comfortable in the situation. Otherwise, none of it makes any sense. And in order to feel that way, I'm allowed to do another vaginal exam, even if it won't necessarily change the course of action. Of course, I always communicate that I'm doing the vaginal exam because it will help me better assess the situation and ask permission. I can't pretend to feel good when I feel like I'm missing something that could somehow help me to better understand the situation. I'm also allowed to tell my colleague that I am uncomfortable with something she's doing.

And, finally, after all those transfers, I had a truly beautiful birth.[1] It was a planned home birth. They called me around 10:30 in the evening or so. I drove over there with my home birth equipment, and things progressed pretty quickly. They had a doula with them because the mother had had a really traumatic first birth. At some point, something really incredible happened. I was sitting next to her, listening to the baby's heartbeat, and suddenly I was able to zoom out and see the whole scene from above. And I thought: Wow. I'm really sitting here as a midwife attending a home birth. How surreal is that? This is exactly what I had hoped for when I started training to become a midwife. And now I'm doing it. It was truly amazing—especially after all those traumatic hospital births. This was such a beautiful moment.

Soon after that, she started pushing a bit during a contraction, and went into her birthing pool. I called my second midwife while I was putting on my gloves. After that, she 'breathed' her baby out. She didn't even have to push. It was exhilarating. At one point I said, "You can let go now." And she said, "I'm scared." So, I told her, "Then go slowly. Trust yourself." I felt like we were deeply connected. I had my hand lightly on the baby's head, and with each breath, with each exhalation, the baby filled out my hand more and more. She was hesitant to let go, and that made the baby's head come so slowly—so gently. It was really beautiful. Her older child woke up when he heard the first cries of his brother and came running into the room. It was sublime.

This is where I'm at now. Out-of-hospital birth, like home birth or birth centre work, is always portrayed as so romantic and cozy—like those are the midwives who just love a comfy atmosphere but aren't clinically astute. And then hospital birth is framed as the tough stuff—the midwives who really know what they're doing, who are totally on the ball. And I was like, well, here I am, completely alone, in the middle of the night, responsible for two lives, and am completely aware of the clinical situation—managing it moment by moment AND I'm staying calm and gentle and am able to create this so-called "romantic atmosphere." And I thought—what a funny contradiction. Those two things don't cancel each other out. Like, this really flips the script.

In this final interview, Amelia once again shows signs of having reached the stage of proficient practitioner. Benner (1984) describes the proficient practitioner as capable of perceiving situations as wholes, which Amelia is clearly able to do in these stories. Benner (1984) writes:

Because of the experience-based ability to recognize whole situations, the proficient nurse can now recognise when the expected normal picture does not present itself…The holistic understanding of the proficient nurse improves his or her decision making. Decision making is less laboured since the nurse has a perspective about which of the many attributes and aspects present are the important ones.

(p. 405)

Amelia knew exactly what to do, carrying out each step on her own. Her experience during the emergency transfer exemplifies what Dreyfus refers to as skilled coping. In that moment, she was no longer relying on explicit rules (she did not have to read a list) or conscious problem-solving. Instead, her actions emerged from an embodied fluency, an intuitive responsiveness shaped by past experiences and critical reflection. Dreyfus contends that expertise necessitates the ability to respond meaningfully without stepping outside the flow of practice, which Amelia was clearly able to do.

Amelia's story reveals how becoming the midwife she dreamed of becoming was a matter of physiological safety, emotional presence, and relational attunement, in addition to the development of clinical skills. Polyvagal Theory helps us see that this transformation was made possible by a context in which her nervous system could shift out of defence and into connection. In the birth centre, she no longer had to brace herself against judgement or suppression; instead, she could get oriented to working in a supportive team at her own pace, learning to trust herself while offering trust to others. Her sense of self as a midwife became possible through a relational field that supported a calm disposition, responsiveness, and co-regulation. It is this very capacity, to act with clarity in uncertainty while maintaining presence, that marks her becoming a skilled, fully present midwife in the profession she had only imagined was possible.

Questions for reflection

1 Amelia's story reveals how clinical confidence and relational presence can develop in a supportive environment. What elements in your current or past learning environments have made you feel safe (or unsafe) and how has this affected your ability to learn?

2 Polyvagal Theory suggests that safety is a prerequisite for connection. Can you recall a clinical situation where your nervous system was in a state of calm versus a state of stress? How did this impact your ability to be present with clients?

3 Amelia gradually internalises responsibility and clinical judgement. At what point did, or might you, begin to see yourself as equally responsible in a birth scenario? What supported or inhibited that shift?

4 Amelia experiences a shift from rigidly following scripts to trusting her own voice and presence. How do you navigate the tension between following guidelines and developing your own clinical style?

5 Amelia comes to a moment of self-recognition: "I'm really doing this. I'm a midwife." What does your version of that moment look or feel like? What does "becoming the midwife you dream of becoming" mean for you?

Note

1 This story is adapted from an earlier version published in Stone, N. I., Thomson, G., & Tegethoff, D. (2023, Dec 27). 'Bringing forth' skills and knowledge of newly qualified midwives in free-standing birth centres: A hermeneutic phenomenological study. *J Adv Nurs*, *80*(8), 3309–3322. https://doi.org/10.1111/jan.16029 Readers interested in a more detailed discussion can refer to that paper.

References

Benner, P. (1984). *From Novice to Expert, Excellence and Power in Clinical Nursing Practice*. Prentice Hall.

Dreyfus, H. L. (2014). *Skillful Coping Essays on the Phenomenology of Everyday Perception and Action* (M. A. Wrathall, Ed.). Oxford University Press.

Dreyfus, H. L., & Dreyfus, S. E. (2005). Expertise in real world contexts. *OS, 26*(5), 777–792. https://doi.org/10.1177/0170840605053102

Dreyfus, S. E. (1981). *Four Models v Human Situational Understanding: Inherent Limitations on the Modelling of Business Expertise*. https://apps.dtic.mil/sti/pdfs/ADA097468.pdf

Dreyfus, S. E., & Dreyfus, H. L. (1980). *A Five-Stage Model of Mental Activities Involved in Directed Skill Acquisition*. https://apps.dtic.mil/dtic/tr/fulltext/u2/a084551.pdf

Porges, S. W. (2011). *The Polyvagal Theory: Neurophysiological Foundations of Emotions, Attachment, Communication, and Self-Regulation* (1st ed.). W. W. Norton.

Porges, S. W. (2022). Polyvagal theory: A science of safety. *Front Integr Neurosci, 16*, 871227. https://doi.org/10.3389/fnint.2022.871227

Stone, N. I., Thomson, G., & Tegethoff, D. (2023, Dec 27). 'Bringing forth' skills and knowledge of newly qualified midwives in free-standing birth centres: A hermeneutic phenomenological study. *J Adv Nurs*, *80*(8), 3309–3322. https://doi.org/10.1111/jan.16029

14

RECLAIMING PRESENCE

Many midwives describe feeling drawn to the relational depth of caring for labouring and birthing women, which they regard as central to midwifery practice (Doherty, 2010; Nilsson et al., 2019; Simonds et al., 2007). However, for students, the structure of clinical training often leaves little room for relational care. Most participants in this study described their clinical placements as stressful and at odds with their expectations, suggesting the need to reflect on how learning environments can better support students. While some did recall moments of connection and affirmation, many shared stories of situations that felt misaligned with their hopes and aspirations. This reflects a broader issue in midwifery education, where students do not feel valued and struggle to process the events they witness, at times becoming emotionally overwhelmed (Coldridge & Davies, 2017).

A positive learning and work environment supports more than skill acquisition; it cultivates well-being. When students and newly qualified midwives encounter cues of belonging and respect, their autonomic nervous systems register safety, enabling social engagement (Porges, 2022). In such states, shame and withdrawal are less likely, and students and early career midwives are better able to absorb knowledge, connect with others, and grow in confidence. A supportive environment also strengthens the alignment between personal values and professional practice, fostering what Heidegger (1971) calls dwelling rather than the experience of alienation or ontological homelessness.

In contrast, adapting to dysfunctional work settings and poor relationships with colleagues by compromising one's values, while often a pragmatic adjustment, is a defensive response that slowly erodes one's own capacity to dwell and engage with others (Porges, 2011). Over time, such compromises may diminish a student or newly qualified midwife's capacity to remain present in ways that sustain meaningful care, not only affecting how she practices, but how she experiences herself

DOI: 10.4324/9781003591306-14

in the role. While there are many reasons to choose working in a free-standing birth centre or offering home birth services as a newly qualified midwife, perhaps a longing for connection and neurophysiological safety, for themselves and for the women and families they care for, is a message we should not overlook. I believe that it gestures towards more than environment; it is a yearning for an ontological home, and the possibility of finding a safe place within oneself to extend to others, essential to offering ethical, relational care.

Mentorship plays an important role in easing the transition from student to newly qualified midwife. When supportive colleagues model relational practice, this is often experienced as transformative. In the free-standing birth centres, mentorship provided a buffer against the disorienting remnants of clinical training, offering not only practical guidance but also providing cues of safety and belonging. By acknowledging uncertainty and allowing time for gradual growth, mentors created an environment where newly qualified midwives could cultivate both skills and confidence. Such support reinforced professional values, facilitating the capacity to be present. In cultivating the confidence to grow professionally, newly qualified midwives were able to step into the role they had envisioned for themselves.

Learning to dwell: Developing relational perception in midwifery practice

To facilitate social engagement and relational care, the newly qualified midwives first needed to slow down and experience time as a gift given for connection. Observing the interactions between their experienced colleagues and their clients opened up novel ways of perceiving space, where issues that "hung in the air" could be addressed. Witnessing empathic communication and taking note of their colleagues' words and body language helped them attune differently to clients than they had in their clinical practice. These were all first steps in learning to see the whole.

Midwifery education, like all medical training, includes comprehensive instruction in anatomy, physiology, and pathophysiology, as well as theoretical constructs intended to guide practice. These constructs function as cognitive boundaries, shaping how associations are formed, how diagnoses are made, and how clinical decisions are justified. In many hospital labour wards, clinical interactions are brief. Practitioners often meet birthing women for the first time during labour, and assessment is typically based on data collected via technological monitoring, as well as a short verbal account. This approach to care narrows focus, stripping labour and birth from the broader context of a woman's life. Used in isolation, technological readings tend to flatten lived experience into discrete variables, separating it from the relational and narrative dimensions that also shape and add meaning to what is transpiring.

For the newly qualified midwives, learning to "see" differently meant engaging senses beyond vision to gather layers of information that are unavailable to the eyes, giving life to information that otherwise appears superficial and flat. Donna Haraway (1988) writes that vision is neither neutral nor passive. There is no such thing as a purely objective or unmediated view. The use of modern visual technologies always involves perspective, translation, and interpretation. Every way of seeing and every image reflects a specific standpoint that organises the world in a specific way. Providing care that goes beyond what eyes can see and machines can measure requires auditory and tactile skills to perceive what is hidden by limited perception and constructs that explain only part of reality.

In the free-standing birth centres, clinical care remained central, but the process of gathering information was multi-dimensional. Midwives combined objective data with attunement to client needs, opening the possibility of shifting into Kairos time. Emotions were not background noise that needed to be suppressed, but meaningful signals shaping each encounter. Through abdominal palpation, they established a kinetic relationship with the unborn baby, sensing position, mobility, and responsiveness of the baby (haptic perception), as well as registering the temperature of their client's skin, the consistency of her tissues, and the reactivity and readiness of the uterus, all forms of tactile listening. Lastly, they became aware of the atmosphere, the unspoken mood in the room, and their own contribution to calmness, joy, and fear.

Through the practice of documenting births as stories, newly qualified midwives began to recognise the nuance and impact of dialogue, interaction, activity, and emotions. These were not only forensic records; they became interpretive acts, revealing the labour dynamic, as well as the relationship dynamics. With this documentation, the midwives came to understand care as relationally co-constructed, unfolding in presence. These dimensions gave depth and shape to their practice, allowing them to dwell more fully with those in their care.

Learning to dwell with clients and colleagues required time, trust, and deep reflection. Over time, the newly qualified midwives began to rely less on theoretical constructs to explain the whole, instead leaning into the ambiguity and complexity of each birth. This was not an abandonment of clinical knowledge but a reconfiguration of how that knowledge was used. During their orientation, they began to see differently, make new associations, notice subtler details, and reorient their perspective towards birth and women's capacity to give birth.

Care as story

Midwives' birth stories differ from women's birth stories. Women tell their birth story as a singular event, often shaped by the memory of contractions, pain, and the physical effort of bringing a child into the world. Midwives, by contrast, accumulate many birth stories, each one added to the next, forming a repertoire that continually shapes their practice and their presence. They draw on these stories to cultivate self-trust and professional identity, carried forward by the dynamic of each lived experience. Their stories—told and retold, shared with researchers and colleagues, or replayed inwardly—offer a way to reflect on and understand their significance for practice.

Midwives enter the lives of women and families midstream, and, when they leave, their shared experiences continue to ripple outward in the lives of those they care for, as well as in their own. Relational care can transform the story of birth into a story of *us*, demonstrating the vital role of relationship in supporting physiological processes. Some births leave a deeper imprint than others, moments that become personal and professional turning points. Any one moment, taken alone, might seem ordinary, yet together, they disclose the deeper meaning of relational practice.

Relational care is not bound by setting. Even within the highly structured environment of a hospital, it is possible to be guided by a client's innate, embodied knowledge and allow her labour to progress in its own time. While I was finishing this last chapter, I experienced such a connection during a busy shift in the hospital where I work. The woman I was caring for was 41 + 1 weeks pregnant, admitted the day before for a planned induction due to a non-reassuring fetal heart tracing and oligohydramnios (low amniotic fluid volume). We met early in the morning at the beginning of my 12-hour shift for her first CTG of the day. That initial tracing was also non-reassuring, with a bradycardia during a strong contraction. I palpated her uterus, discovered that her baby was in an occiput-posterior position, and interpreted the bradycardia as a vagal response to pressure on the large fontanelle. Though her cervix was only 2 cm dilated, that reaction told me that the contractions had significant strength.

The attending physician suggested induction, which our client declined. I asked her what she thought should happen next instead. She told me that she simply needed more time to allow her contractions to get stronger and preferred to wait. She was certain that her labour would progress on its own. I believed her. Throughout the day, she alternated between periods of contractions every five to seven minutes and periods of rest, in which she was able to sleep. I attended to her needs, checking in regularly to monitor the baby's heartbeat, but otherwise did not disturb her. Witnessing her labour dynamic reminded me of an interview that I conducted with a home birth midwife in France more than 20 years ago, an interview I often recall when caring for a woman with this labour pattern. She described an "occiput-posterior labour dynamic" (when the baby's back is turned towards the woman's spine): contractions come for an hour or two, followed by periods of rest, until, at some point, the labour dynamic accelerates, and the woman gives birth quickly. I could hear the voice of that midwife telling me this story years before as I watched my client's labour unfold.

She stayed in the labour and delivery ward, where all subsequent CTGs were normal. We had the whole day to connect and build a trusting relationship. At 5 pm, her contractions grew stronger and were painful for the first time that day. She did not want further vaginal examinations, nor did she want artificial rupture of the membranes, which I gladly respected. Her baby was still in an occiput-posterior position, evident from frontal kicks on both sides of her abdomen. She preferred an upright kneeling position, and I followed her lead. I had been attuned to her throughout the day, and in those moments, felt joy witnessing her labour unfold on her own terms. At 6 pm, neither of us expected she would give birth before my shift ended at 7 pm; however, both of us were pleased she had the time and space to go into labour without an induction. After briefly leaving the room to attend to another labouring woman, she called me back into the room at 6:10. At 6:20, her membranes ruptured spontaneously, and at 6:30, she birthed her baby, kneeling and using only her breath to birth his head, followed by a single push to complete the birth. I was in awe of her courage, patience, and strength.

As a midwife who has worked in many settings, I treasure the stories of my colleagues and those entrusted to me in interviews. These stories become resources for research and practice, shaping how I interpret and understand birth, one labour at a time. Stories carry experience across time and place, making it possible for midwives to practice together, even after years have passed. These stories remind us that midwifery knowledge lives in stories of care, told and retold. They are how we remember what matters, how we recognise patterns, and how we keep alive the relational essence of our profession. Sharing these stories honours the past, as well as shaping the future, cultivating the presence that sustains ethical, relational care in every setting. In this way, the story is not only memory but method, a way of dwelling together, guiding us towards presence at every birth.

References

Coldridge, L., & Davies, S. (2017, Feb). "Am I too emotional for this job?" An exploration of student midwives' experiences of coping with traumatic events in the labour ward. *Midwifery, 45*, 1–6. https://doi.org/10.1016/j.midw.2016.11.008

Doherty, M. E. (2010, Mar-Apr). Voices of midwives: A tapestry of challenges and blessings. *MCN Am J Matern Child Nurs, 35*(2), 96–101. https://doi.org/10.1097/NMC.0b013e3181caea9f

Haraway, D. (1988). Situated knowledges: The science question in feminism and the privilege of partial perspective. *FS, 14*(3), 575–599. https://links.jstor.org/sici?sici=0046-3663%28198823%2914%3A3%3C575%3ASKTSQI%3E2.0.CO%3B2-M

Heidegger, M. (1971). *Poetry, Language, Thought* (1st ed.). Harper & Row.

Nilsson, C., Olafsdottir, O. A., Lundgren, I., Berg, M., & Dellenborg, L. (2019, Dec). Midwives' care on a labour ward prior to the introduction of a midwifery model of care: A field of tension. *Int J Qual Stud Health Well-being, 14*(1), 1593037. https://doi.org/10.1080/17482631.2019.1593037

Porges, S. W. (2011). *The Polyvagal Theory: Neurophysiological Foundations of Emotions, Attachment, Communication, and Self-Regulation* (1st ed.). W. W. Norton.

Porges, S. W. (2022). Polyvagal theory: A science of safety. *Front Integr Neurosci, 16*, 871227. https://doi.org/10.3389/fnint.2022.871227

Simonds, W., Rothman, B. K., & Norman, B. M. (2007). *Laboring on: Birth in Transition in the United States*. Routledge. Table of contents only. https://www.loc.gov/catdir/toc/ecip075/2006028290.html

For Product Safety Concerns and Information please contact our EU
representative GPSR@taylorandfrancis.com
Taylor & Francis Verlag GmbH, Kaufingerstraße 24, 80331 München, Germany

www.ingramcontent.com/pod-product-compliance
Lightning Source LLC
Chambersburg PA
CBHW060316220326
41598CB00027B/4347